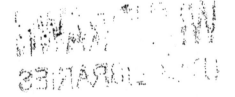

Insects and disease

Insects and disease

Keith R Snow Ph D

Lecturer in Biological Science
North East London Polytechnic

London: Routledge & Kegan Paul

*First published in 1974
by Routledge & Kegan Paul Ltd
Broadway House, 68–74 Carter Lane,
London EC4V 5EL
Filmset and printed by BAS Printers Limited,
Wallop, Hampshire*
© *Keith R. Snow 1974*
*No part of this book may be reproduced in
any form without permission from the
publisher, except for the quotation of brief
passages in criticism*

*ISBN 0 7100 7706 8 (c)
ISBN 0 7100 7707 6 (p)*

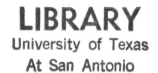

To Amanda and Samantha

Contents

Preface

Few people would question the importance of insects in the spread
of disease to man and domesticated animals, for they have long
been known to transmit such killer diseases as malaria, sleeping
sickness and plague. It is therefore not surprising that a great deal
has been written about them and the pathogens that they carry.

This book is an attempt to bring together the more important
aspects of the biology of both the insect vectors and the disease-
producing organisms. It is in no way intended to be a reference
book but it is an introduction to the subject which may at the same
time arouse the interest and curiosity of the reader in this aspect
of parasitology.

The book is divided into two main parts, the first of which deals
with the insects that cause disease either directly by their presence
or by introducing organisms into an animal. The second part is
devoted to the pathogens themselves and contains accounts on all
of the major insect-borne species. Although the subject matter has
been divided in this manner, purely for ease of reference, an effort
has been made to correlate the biology of the insect with that of
the pathogen.

It is hoped that the book will prove useful to those studying for
qualifications in parasitology, entomology and general zoology at
degree or equivalent standard as well as for persons with a desire
to supplement their present knowledge in this sphere.

Accompanying the text are a large number of diagrams which
have been drawn specially for this book by the author. They are
based on actual specimens, personal observations and data
assembled from the scientific literature.

I should like to express my sincere thanks to Professor D. R.

Arthur and Dr F. E. G. Cox for their comments and suggestions and to Dr J. M. Watson for reading the chapters on the pathogens. Miss Pat Stone, B.Pharm., M.P.S., made a useful contribution to the book with her valuable help concerning the drugs used in the treatment of the diseases carried by insects. Finally, I am most grateful to Mrs Janet Bunyard for her willing help in typing the manuscript in its final as well as its numerous draft forms.

1

Introduction

Insects are members of the phylum Arthropoda which contains a vast assemblage of forms sharing certain common features, many of which are either a direct consequence of, or relate to, the possession of a chitinous exoskeleton. A number of fairly distinct evolutionary lines can be recognized within the Arthropoda, the insects being just one of these. Fig. 1 shows the main classes of arthropodan invertebrates together with their diagnostic characteristics, and should serve to facilitate their recognition and differentiation from one another.

The insectan body is composed of a head, thorax and abdomen, with a pair of legs located on each of the three thoracic segments. Most insects can fly and have two pairs of wings articulating with the second and third thoracic segments. In the majority of cases there are no appendages on the abdomen apart from the accessory reproductive structures. Respiration in insects is usually by means of a tracheal system and the life cycle is often complex showing a distinct metamorphosis.

The head
The insectan head is a more or less spherical capsule joined to the thorax by means of a flexible membranous neck. It bears the eyes, which may be classed as either compound or simple (Fig. 2 A), the mouthparts and the antennae, which typically consist of a basal scape, a pedicel, a meriston and a flagellum of many divisions (Fig. 2 C).

The pattern of the antenna varies considerably throughout the insects and there may, in addition, be sexual dimorphism. In

1

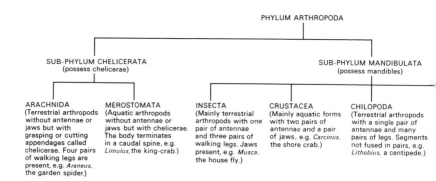

Figure 1 The main classes of arthropods and their characteristics.

mosquitoes, for example, the flagellum bears a number of long setae. In the male the antenna is thickly bristled and known as plumose, while in females it is only slightly hairy and called pilose. In some groups of insects there is an additional sidebranch of the antenna called the arista.

The mouthparts of disease-transmitting insects

The food and feeding habits of insects are extremely varied and, as we might expect, their mouthparts have become adapted to suit their individual diets. Even though the patterns of insect mouthparts are extremely diverse it is possible to refer them to a basic pattern and to speculate on the ways in which they have evolved. It is usually believed that the basic method of feeding is that of biting and chewing, and it is thus thought that insects like the locust and cockroach will show us the basic mouthpart arrangement (Fig. 2).

As is typical of insects, the locust and cockroach have a head composed of six embryonic segments, some of which have appendages as indicated in Table 1.

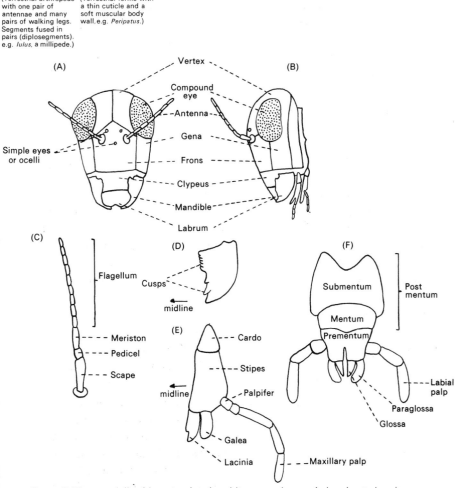

DIPLOPODA
(Terrestrial arthropods
with one pair of
antennae and many
pairs of walking legs.
Segments fused in
pairs (diplosegments).
e.g. *Iulus,* a millipede.)

ONYCHOPHORA
(Terrestrial forms with
a thin cuticle and a
soft muscular body
wall, e.g. *Peripatus.*)

(A)

(B)

Vertex

Compound
eye

Antenna

Gena

Simple eyes
or ocelli

Frons

Clypeus

Mandible

Labrum

(C)

Flagellum

Cusps

midline

(D)

(F)

Submentum

Post
mentum

Mentum

Prementum

Meriston

(E)

Cardo

Pedicel

Scape

Stipes

midline

Palpifer

Labial
palp

Paraglossa

Glossa

Galea

Lacinia

Maxillary palp

Figure 2 The generalized insectan head and its appendages : A, head anterior view ;
B, head lateral view ; C, antenna ; D, mandible ; E, maxilla ; F, labium.

Table 1 The head segments of an insect

Segment		Adult appendage
1	preantennal	none
2	antennal	antenna
3	intercalary	none
4	mandibular	mandible
5	maxillary	maxilla
6	labial	labium

In those insects where the emphasis is on chewing and biting the mandibles are large and denticulate. Behind the mandibles are the paired maxillae, each of which is joined to the head by means of a basal cardo (pl. cardines). This articulates with the stipes (pl. stipites) which carries a palp-bearing sclerite, the palpifer, and distally two podomeres, an inner lacinia and an outer galea. The labium is found behind the other mouthparts and is formed by the fusion of the appendages of the last head segment. It consists of a basal postmentum equivalent to the fused cardines of the maxilla and a prementum formed from the fused stipites. The prementum bears the labial palps and, internally, the ligulae. Each ligula is composed of two lobes, the median glossa and the lateral paraglossa.

Additional to the segmental appendages there are two other structures which contribute to the mouthparts. These are the labrum which arises from a head plate, the clypeus, in front of the mouth, and the hypopharynx which in many insects bears the opening of the salivary duct. A sensory epipharynx is also present, which in some insects is closely associated with the labrum.

Of the insects which spread disease to man and other animals the biting lice have mouthparts which resemble the basic pattern most closely. This is because they use their mandibles to bite off short lengths of hair and feather. However, their other mouthparts are severely modified, for the labium and maxillae are not involved in feeding to any extent while the labrum has the role of pushing the food into the mouth.

When we look at the remainder of the ectoparasitic insects we find that modifications have occurred in the mouthparts to adapt the adults to a blood or tissue fluid diet. In these insects the mouthparts are formed into a proboscis which is capable of penetrating the skin of the host animal and removing fluids from it. The proboscis has evolved several times in a number of different groups of insect and has been formed in various ways.

In general it is possible to consider changes in the mouthparts as being due to either the modification or the loss of a component part (Table 2). Thus in the fleas the mandibles have been lost and the remaining mouthparts modified to form the proboscis, with penetration being effected by the laciniae of the maxillae which are armed with numerous fine teeth. Mandibles have also been lost by most adult sucking lice (Anoplura), and in this case the labium is modified as the main organ of penetration.

Table 2 The major mouthpart modifications shown by parasitic insects

Modification	Insect
maxillae and mandibles developed for penetration	mosquitoes, sandflies, midges, blackflies, tabanids and bugs
labium modified for penetration; mandibles absent	tsetse flies, stable flies, keds and sucking lice
maxillary laciniae used for penetration; mandibles absent	fleas
mandibles alone developed for cutting	biting lice
mouthparts absent	bot flies and warble flies

The labium is also modified in a number of other insects such as the keds, stable flies (*Stomoxys*) and tsetse flies (*Glossina*). In the latter case only maxillary palps, labrum, hypopharynx and labium are present, with the tip of the labium being heavily armed with teeth and rasping plates. An evolutionary series may be demonstrated using the genera *Musca, Stomoxys* and *Glossina* as examples (Fig. 3). The first of these contains, in the main, non-parasitic members which feed on free fluids and particles which they rasp from solid material, while members of the other two genera are ectoparasitic and use their labellar armature to pierce the skin of their host.

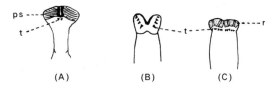

(A)   (B)   (C)

Figure 3 Modification of the labellar lobes of various dipterans. In *Musca domestica* (A) the lobes are soft and equipped with pseudotracheae (ps) used for imbibing fluids. However, there are a number of small plates called prestomal teeth (t) present. In *Musca crassirostris* (not shown) the teeth are larger and the insects can cut skin to obtain blood which they then feed upon using their pseudotracheae. In *Stomoxys calcitrans* (B) the labella are hard and the teeth more fully developed, while in *Glossina palpalis* (C) the hardened and toothed labella are equipped with rasping plates (r) which aid penetration.

The importance of the mandibles, even in insects with a proboscis, can be seen in the blackflies, biting midges and tabanid flies. All three have short proboscides with the well-developed scissor (or blade)-like mandibles having a major role in penetration. Mosquitoes, sandflies and bugs also employ the mandibles in penetration, but in these insects the maxillae are also important and both of these mouthparts are drawn out to form stylets.

The thorax and abdomen
Three segments, the pro-, meso- and metathorax, make up the insectan *thorax*, each of which bears a pair of walking legs

composed of six divisions: coxa, trochanter, femur, tibia, tarsus and pretarsus. Additionally, the mesothorax (second segment) and the metathorax (third segment) bear wings, which are flat membranous processes arising from between the tergal and the pleural plates of the body (Fig. 4). Each wing is supported by a framework of

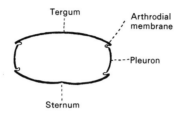

Figure 4 Transverse section through the body of an arthropod to show the arrangement of the segmental plates.

longitudinal and transverse cuticular thickenings called veins, the number and arrangement of which is of taxonomic importance. A few groups of insects (e.g. fleas, lice and keds) have secondarily lost their wings, a phenomenon which is connected with their more or less permanent ectoparasitic way of life.

Eleven segments and a terminal telson form the *abdomen*, not all of which are necessarily visible. The eighth and ninth segments in the female and the ninth only in the male carry the external genitalia, and from the eleventh segment arise the sensory cerci. In the male the external genitalia take the form of a median intromittent organ or aedaegus and organs to clasp the female during mating. The external genitalia of the female often form an ovipositor used in egg-laying.

Very few of the internal features of insects need concern us here, except for the alimentary canal. In most insects three gut regions can be recognized: the foregut, or stomodaeum; the midgut, or mesenteron; and the hindgut, or proctodaeum. Further subdivisions of these sections can be made, as shown in Fig. 5.

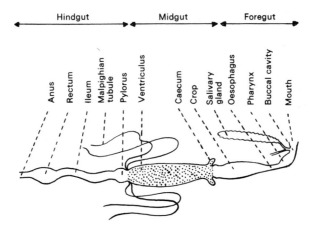

Figure 5 The gut regions of a typical insect.

Immature stages and life histories

The life cycle of an insect is composed of a number of distinct stages, or instars, each of which is separated from the next by an ecdysis, or moult. The stage which hatches from the egg is the *larva*, and in apterygote and hemimetabolous insects there is a gradual change, more marked in the latter, from the larva to the adult instar. In holometabolous insects, on the other hand, the larva is unlike the adult and the change from one to the other takes place in an intervening stage known as the *pupa*. Such a life history permits considerable morphological differences to occur between the larva and adult such that the two instars can be adapted for life in quite different habitats.

A number of different types of larvae and pupae can be recognized. With regard to the larvae, four major categories have been demonstrated.

1 *Nymph*   The larva of hemimetabolous and apterygote insects which closely resembles the adult.

2 *Oligopod larva*   Possesses six legs (hexapod) and found in, for example, the Neuroptera and Coleoptera.

3 *Polypod larva*   With six walking legs and few to numerous
auxillary supporting legs (prolegs), as in, for example, the
Lepidoptera.

4 *Apod larva*   These lack legs and are of three types:
    eucephalous—with a well-developed head capsule; found in
    most Nematocera (Diptera).
    hemicephalous—with a reduced head capsule which can be
    retracted into the thorax; found in the Brachycera (Diptera).
    acephalous—with no head capsule; found in the Cyclorrhapha
    (Diptera).

One of two types of pupae may develop from the larval stage in
holometabolous insects. In, for example, the Coleoptera,
Siphonaptera, cyclorrhaphan and brachyceran dipterans the
appendages of the developing adult are free of the body of the
pupa, a condition described as *exarate*. In contrast to this,
however, nematoceran dipterans and most Lepidoptera exhibit a
condition in which the legs adhere to the pupal body. This type of
pupa is said to be *obtectate*.

Classification of the insects causing important diseases
Of about thirty orders of insects only five require detailed mention
here, as these alone are responsible for the spread of the majority of
diseases to man and domesticated animals. A complete list of the
orders of insects may be found in appendix I of this book.

1 *Order Diptera*   These possess one pair of wings on the
mesothorax only.

Suborder 1 Nematocera   The antennae of adults are longer than
    the combined length of the head and thorax and are
    composed of more than eight divisions. The antenna
    does not possess an arista. Larva have well-developed
    mandibles and pupae are obtectate.

Family Simuliidae (blackflies)   Small flies, between 1 and 5 mm in length, with a humped thorax and a short proboscis. Eggs are laid below the surface of running water. Larvae possess a proleg near the anterior end (e.g. *Simulium*).

Family Psychodidae (sandflies)   Small, moth-like flies rarely more than 4 mm in length in which the antennae are of sixteen divisions and the bodies and wings are covered with hair-like processes. Eggs are laid in moist places and hatch into legless larvae (e.g. *Phlebotomus*).

Family Culicidae (mosquitoes)   Slender flies with spherical heads and elongated legs. The flagella of the antennae consist of thirteen or fourteen divisions and are plumose in males and pilose in females. The proboscis is long and slender and the long, narrow wings have leaf-like scales along their margins and on the veins. The thorax is subtriangular in shape and the abdomen is elongated. Larvae and pupae are aquatic and characteristic (e.g. *Aedes, Anopheles, Culex*).

Family Ceratopogonidae (biting midges)   Minute flies usually less than 3 mm in length with a humped thorax and a short proboscis. The antennae are long and are plumose in males and pilose in females. The wings are covered in hair-like structures and lack scales. Eggs are laid in water and the larva, which is aquatic or semi-aquatic, possesses three posterior retractile anal gills (e.g. *Culicoides*).

Suborder 2   Brachycera   The antennae are shorter than the thorax and are composed of less than six divisions. An arista may be present as part of the antenna.

Family Tabanidae (horseflies)   Stout flies with large heads and an antenna of two short basal divisions and a third which is elongated and subdivided. The wing venation is characteristic (e.g. *Chrysops, Tabanus*).

Suborder 3   Cyclorrhapha   The antennae possess three divisions and an arista, and the abdomen usually has less than seven visible segments. On the head there is a U-shaped ridge which is the characteristic ptilinal suture (see page 53).

Family Gasterophilidae (bot flies)   Adult flies are large and hairy with rudimentary mouthparts and do not feed. The eggs are usually laid on an animal which is to be parasitized by the larval stage. The larvae are located in the gut of mammals and leave the host to pupate (e.g. *Gasterophilus*).

Family Oestridae (warble flies)   As for the family Gasterophilidae except that the larvae are parasitic in or under the skin of various animals or within a body cavity (e.g. *Oestrus, Hypoderma*).

Family Muscidae (house flies, tsetse flies, etc.)   Small to medium sized flies, some of which have mouthparts adapted for piercing skin. The wing is characteristic in that the median wing vein (see b in Fig. 51) is either parallel to the fused fourth and fifth radial veins (see a in Fig. 51) or curves towards it (e.g. *Musca, Glossina, Stomoxys*).

Family Calliphoridae (blowflies, flesh flies)   Large flies with a cleft on the anterior margin of the second antennal division (shared with Muscidae) and with a poorly developed post-scutellum. They can be differentiated from muscids by the presence of bristles on the hypopleuron of the thorax (Fig. 6) (e.g. *Calliphora, Chrysomyia*).

Family Hippoboscidae (louse flies, keds)   Flies with a dorso-ventrally compressed body and with legs possessing claws for attachment to the host. The antennae are of one division only and lie within a depression in the head. Wings may be present or absent. All forms are viviparous (e.g. *Hippobosca, Melophagus*).

Anterior ◄──────

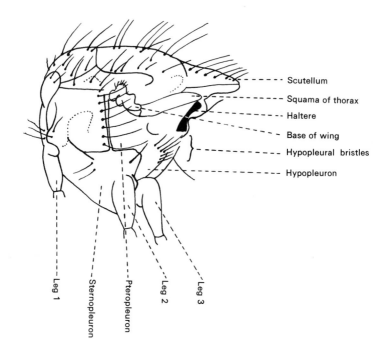

Figure 6 Thorax of a calliphorid fly, lateral view.

2 *Order Hemiptera*   These are bugs with piercing and suctorial
mouthparts. The forewings either have a thickened basal region
and a distal membranous portion or are entirely membranous. The
hindwings are always completely membranous.

Suborder 1   *Homoptera*   The forewings are completely
             membranous and the labium of the proboscis
             originates far back on the head.

Suborder 2   *Heteroptera*   The forewings have a thickened basal
             region (hemelytra) and the labium originates
             anteriorly on the head.

Family Reduviidae (Triatomidae) (assassin bugs)
Medium to large bugs in which the antennae are long
and filamentous and the labium is of three divisions
(e.g. *Triatoma, Rhodnius*).
Family Cimicidae (bed-bugs)   Ovoid, dorso-ventrally
flattened bugs with vestigial hemelytra (e.g. *Cimex*).

3 *Order Siphonaptera (Aphaniptera)* (fleas)   These are small,
wingless, laterally compressed insects. The adults have piercing and
suctorial mouthparts and elongated, clawed legs for jumping and
attachment. The larvae are vermiform and non-parasitic (e.g. *Pulex,
Ctenocephalides*).

4 *Order Anoplura (Siphunculata)* (sucking lice)   These insects
have mouthparts adapted for piercing skin and sucking the body
fluids of their mammalian host. Wings are absent and the thoracic
segments are fused. Each leg terminates in a single, curved claw
(e.g. *Pediculus, Haematopinus*).

5 *Order Mallophaga* (biting lice)   These small, wingless insects
have biting mouthparts and legs with one or two claws. The meso-
and metathorax are often fused but the prothorax is free. They are
ectoparasites of birds and mammals (e.g. *Menopon, Columbicola*).

Parasites and vectors
Because of the high density of animal populations and their need
for similar environmental conditions it is inevitable that animals will
come into contact with one another. This coming together of
animals, whether they be of similar or different species, is termed
animal association. Varying degrees of association exist: for
example, animals of the same species may be solitary for most of
their lives and associate during mating only, or, on the other hand,
they may be gregarious and live together continuously. Animals of
different species may, by sharing the same ecological habitat, be
mere neighbours and quite independent of one another, or they

may be partly reliant on one another, or one or both may be completely dependent on the other. A fuller classification of the types of association is given in Fig. 7.

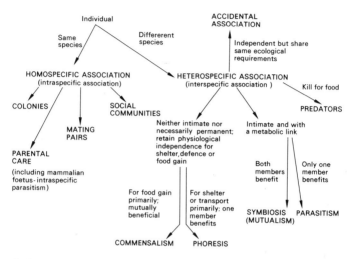

Figure 7 Categories of animal association.

In the present text we are concerned with both the insects and their pathogens as parasites, and it is essential that the term parasitism be well defined in order to differentiate it from other heterospecific associations. However, before an attempt at definition is made, it is perhaps essential to point out that all of the categories are made by man for the use of man and that, although convenient, they do not represent watertight compartments. Intermediate types and exceptions to the definitions as stated must therefore be expected and recognized as such.

It is most important to consider parasitism as being a way of life, that is to say a method of obtaining both food and other environmental needs. Many definitions of parasitism emphasize the harmful effects of the parasite on its host, a point no doubt made bearing in mind the detrimental effects of parasites on man and his domestic stock. However, in their natural host many parasites cause little or no harm and hence it is more satisfactory to use the factor of the metabolic link between the parasite and its partner in the association as a basis of definition. Thus a parasite may be regarded as a living organism having a physiological relationship with and a metabolic dependence on the tissues of another, larger living organism (called its host) of a different species, such that it gains its nutritional requirements from the host. Other requirements of the parasite (e.g. a suitable environment) may also be provided by the host. As a result of the association the host may be harmed, although the damage may be so slight as to be undetectable.

It is not sufficient merely to define a parasite; we must also define the related categories from which parasites must be differentiated (e.g. predator). Basically, a predator, although obtaining its food from another animal (prey), kills that animal outright. In contrast to this, most parasites do not kill their hosts immediately, although some may do so eventually. In general, parasites are also smaller than their hosts (the lamprey may sometimes be an exception), but this may also be true of some predators like the mongoose, weasel and certain snakes.

Subdivisions of parasitism
It is convenient to divide parasites into those which live on the body surface of their hosts (external parasites, or ectoparasites) and those which live inside their hosts (internal parasites, or endoparasites). Again these categories must be thought of as being useful rather than absolute, for a number of parasites do not fit into this scheme with ease. For example the mange mite, *Sarcoptes*, burrows into the skin surface, so that although it is within the body of its host yet its burrow communicates with the outside. It may also be argued that the lumen of the alimentary canal is, strictly speaking, not inside the body and hence it is feasible to class gut parasites as ectoparasites.

Hosts of endoparasitic animals
Endoparasites may have one or more hosts in a life cycle. The host in which either the adult stage or sexual phase occurs is referred to

as the *definitive* or *final* host and the host in which the larval or juvenile stages occur is called the *intermediate* host. More than one intermediate host, of differing species, may occur in a life cycle, in which case the terms first, second, etc., intermediate hosts are employed.

It is not easy to use the above terminology when describing protozoan parasites, as many of them do not have sexual phases and it is often not possible to equate an adult phase in the life cycle. A different terminology must therefore be employed, and it is usual to simply use the term *host* to describe the vertebrate in which the parasite lives and the term *vector* for the invertebrate which transmits the parasite from one host to another. If the protozoan parasite undergoes development within the vector then the transmission is referred to as cyclical. If no such development occurs then it is called non-cyclical transmission. By convention the use of the term vector is now applied to the transmitting agent of many non-protozoan parasites and implies that the invertebrate actively seeks the vertebrate host and deposits the parasite either into the body of the host or on to its surface.

Part I
Biology of the insects

2

Mosquitoes

Mosquitoes are two-winged flies belonging to the family Culicidae of the dipteran suborder Nematocera. This family contains three subfamilies, only one of which—the Culicinae—is of parasitological importance. The characters utilized in the differential diagnosis of adult members of the three subfamilies are shown in the following key:

1 Flagellum of antenna composed of fourteen divisions; mouth-parts not adapted for piercing and no scales on the wings although small setae may be present   DIXINAE
   Flagellum of antenna composed of thirteen divisions; scales present on the wings although their distribution may be restricted   2
2 Mouthparts short and not adapted for piercing and wing scales on the hind margins only   CHAOBORINAE
   Mouthparts long and adapted for piercing; scales on hind margins of wings and on wing veins—these are the mosquitoes (see Fig. 8)   CULICINAE

Not all of the Culicinae concern the parasitologist, for one group, referred to as the tribe Megarhinini, are exclusively plant-feeders and have a probosis so modified as to be incapable of piercing skin. However, the remaining two tribes, the Culicini and the Anophelini, are of interest and are important as both parasites and vectors of disease. Once again it is necessary to distinguish between members of these tribes, and for this purpose an illustrated key to adult characters is given below and a pictorial guide to features of immature anophelines and culicines is presented as Fig. 9.

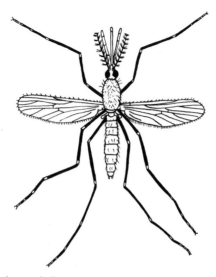

Figure 8 Adult female anopheline mosquito, dorsal view.

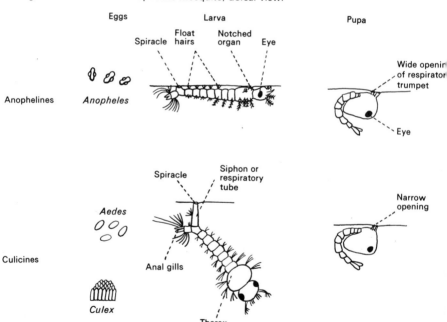

Figure 9 Features of anopheline and culicine immature stages.

1 Abdomen covered with very few scales; the maxillary palps of
   the male and female are long whilst those of the males are
   additionally dilated at their tips; the scutellum of the thorax is
   curved in posterior outline; the body of the insect is held at an
   angle of about 45° to the surface when feeding   ANOPHELINI
   Abdomen completely invested by scales; the female has short
   maxillary palps while those of the male are long but not dilated
   at their tips   2
2 Proboscis rigid but the distal portion is thin and is directed
   ventrally   MEGARHININI
   Proboscis flexible, straight, and of more or less uniform diameter
                                                     CULICINI

   In addition to these characters the body of culicines is held
parallel to the surface when feeding and the posterior margin of the
scutellum is scalloped (Fig. 10).

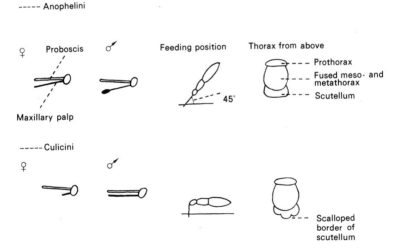

Figure 10 Some features of adult anopheline and culicine mosquitoes.

   All mosquitoes have slender bodies, an elongated piercing
proboscis and a characteristic wing scaling and venation (Fig. 11).
They have two large compound eyes but lack the simple eyes

(ocelli) sometimes found in other insects. The antennae are long
and plumose (thickly bristled) in males and pilose (slightly hairy) in
females. Both the larval and pupal stages are aquatic and active and
differ enormously from the terrestrial adults, thus permitting the
immatures and the imago to be near-perfectly adapted to their own
particular environments.

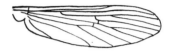

Figure 11 Wing venation of a mosquito.

Mouthparts and feeding

The head of a mosquito bears the mouthparts which are highly
modified for penetration. In the non-feeding insect the elongated
mouthparts fit closely together such that from a lateral view the
labium is the only visible component of the proboscis. The
remaining mouthparts, with the exception of the maxillary palps
which do not contribute to the proboscis, are enclosed within the
hollow of the labium. Distally the labium terminates in a pair of
labellar lobes which are thought to represent the labial palps of
other insects. As seen in cross-section, the labium contains a
forward extension of the haemocoel (blood cavity) of the insect
which is instrumental in the transmission of filarial worms, as is
discussed in chapter 8.

Male mosquitoes may not have a full complement of mouthparts, which is associated with their non-parasitic way of life. In
females the following components are found in addition to the
labium.

The labrum is a strong mouthpart with a pointed apex and is in
the form of a tube with a ventral opening to the outside. As shown
in Fig. 12, the labrum forms the roof and sides of the pre-oral food
canal.

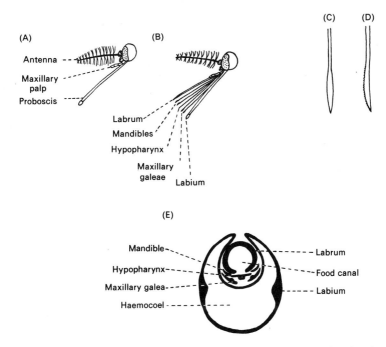

Figure 12 The head and mouthparts of a female mosquito : A, head and proboscis of a non-feeding insect ; B, mouthparts displaced to show the components of the proboscis ; C, distal region of mandible ; D, distal region of a maxillary galea ; E, transverse section through the proboscis.

The flattened hypopharynx is applied to the bottom of the labrum to close its groove, and so completes the canal through which the food materials are drawn. As well as serving this purpose the hypopharynx is itself hollowed to conduct secretions from the salivary glands into the wound during feeding.

Two other mouthparts are also contained within the groove of the labium. They are the slender, spear-like mandibles and the blade-like maxillae which are serrated distally (Fig. 12). It is believed that this part of the maxilla corresponds to the galea of other insects and that the lacinia is lacking. The maxillary palp which is composed of four divisions is, as noted above, not a component of the proboscis of the mosquito.

C

A female mosquito penetrates her host by means of the maxillary blades and the mandibles. The former have saw-like tips and by their alternate movements lacerate the tissues, being aided by the needle-like mandibles. As the mouthparts advance into a skin capillary the labium bends beneath the neck and body (Fig. 13), its

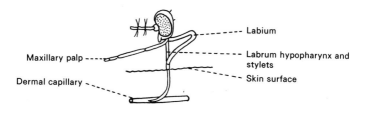

Figure 13 Penetration of a dermal blood vessel by a female mosquito. Note that the maxillary palps and labium do not enter the skin.

tip remaining in contact with the penetrating mouthparts to act as a guide. The proximity of the labium to the skin is of importance in the transmission of nematodes, as noted in chapter 8.

Blood is sucked into the gut by means of two pumps: the cibarial pump formed from the cibarium, a region of the pre-oral food space, and the pharyngeal pump developed from the posterior part of the pharynx (Fig. 14). Both pumps are equipped with external dilator muscles and close by means of their own inherent elasticity. By their rhythmic expansion and contraction the pumps draw fluids up into the pre-oral food canal and finally into the gut. This action is controlled by means of two sphincter muscles which are located close to the posterior regions of each of the pumps.

A third pump is present in mosquitoes in association with the common salivary duct; this helps to expel saliva by way of the hypopharynx. It is equipped with dilator muscles and contracts due to its own elasticity to expel saliva into the tissues and the blood at various stages of penetration. The saliva contains a powerful anticoagulant, and in some species (e.g. *Anopheles maculipennis*) a haemagglutinin is produced by the paired salivary glands, each of which is composed of three lobes. Both have their own separate

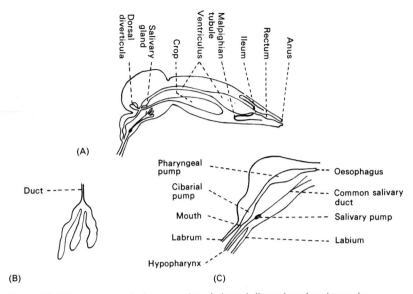

Figure 14 Alimentary canal of a mosquito: A, lateral dissection showing major organs; B, salivary gland; C, longitudinal section through the head to show the pharyngeal and cibarial pumps.

duct, but these eventually join to send a common salivary duct anteriorly to enter the hypopharynx.

The alimentary canal of the mosquito begins with the opening of the pharyngeal pump. This leads to the oesophagus which has three diverticula, one ventral and two dorsal. The ventral pouch is equivalent to the crop of other insects, while the dorsal caecae have no equivalents and are said to be employed in separating air from the imbibed liquids. The oesophagus communicates with the ventriculus which is narrow anteriorly and broader posteriorly, and this in turn leads to the hindgut composed of a short, narrow ileum and an expanded rectum (Fig. 14).

Life histories of mosquitoes

Mosquitoes lay their eggs at various times of the day, for example in the early evening in *Anopheles gambiae* and at about sunset in

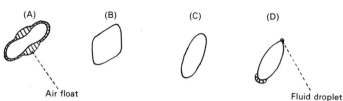

Figure 15 The shapes of mosquito eggs of *Anopheles* (A), *Sabethes* (B), *Aedes* (C), *Culex* (D).

Aedes aegypti. The eggs are generally ovoid, although the shape may be modified considerably. In most *Anopheles* species the outer egg coat (exochorion) is drawn out to produce a lateral frill which is often modified at the sides to give a pair of hollow floats, while the eggs of some *Mansonia* species have one pole drawn out to form a spine or filament. Eggs may be deposited singly or they may, as in *Culex* and some *Mansonia* and *Theobaldia* species, be bound into a group or raft. In many of these latter species the posterior pole of the eggs has a fluid droplet which adds to their buoyancy. A selection of mosquito eggs is shown in Fig. 15.

In most cases the eggs are laid directly into either running or still waters. When they are laid singly they may either be dropped into the water while the female is hovering just above the surface or the female may rest on the surface film of the water as is usual in *Culex* species. A few mosquitoes (e.g. *Aedes* species) may deposit their eggs in floodwater zones such that they are immersed when the water level rises. Running waters (i.e. streams and rivers) are more important habitats of anophelines than culicines, the latter favouring still waters such as pools, swamps, rain puddles, marshes, tree-holes, wells and water held in manufactured articles. The eggs of some species are able to resist desiccation for many months (e.g. the floodwater species mentioned above), and some *Anopheles* species can overwinter in this stage.

Some two or three days after oviposition the egg hatches into the larval instar (Fig. 16). This is an active form which moves either by a jerking of the body, in which case the direction of the locomotion is tail first, or by means of the mouth brushes, which is a consequence of feeding and gives a slow forward movement.

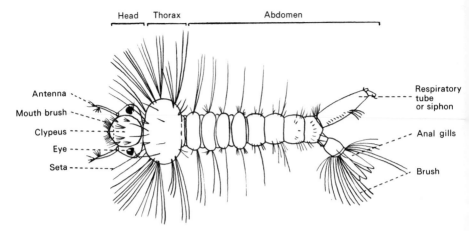

Figure 16 Culicine mosquito larva, dorsal view.

Some larvae, such as those of *Aedes aegypti*, can survive on soluble food exclusively, but in general particulate material is necessary. This may be obtained by rasping at hard materials, scraping algae, ingesting whole large objects such as small crustaceans and other mosquito larvae (this occurs in many *Psorophora* species) or filtering suspended particles from the water (common in anophelines).

As the larvae feed they grow in a characteristic arthropodan manner and moult three times, each of the four intermoult stages being termed a larval instar. Depending on the ambient temperature the time spent in the larval stage will vary, but approximates to about four days. At the onset of winter some species may hibernate as larvae, an example being *Anopheles claviger* from Europe which overwinters buried in the mud at the bottom of the water. Although aquatic, the larvae must breathe air through their respiratory tubes and either come to the surface at intervals or remain there for this purpose. A small amount of gaseous exchange may occur in solution through the body surface. So-called 'anal gills' are present, but these are for the purpose of osmoregulation and not for respiration.

Eventually the larva moults to the pupal stage (Fig. 17) which

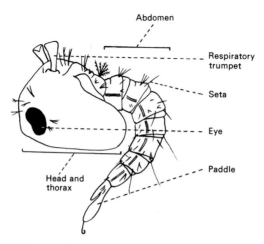

Figure 17 Anopheline pupa, lateral view.

has considerable powers of locomotion by flexion of the abdomen aided by a pair of paddles on the eighth segment. Such movement is probably of great importance as far as survival is concerned. Once again the pupa is an air-breather and has a pair of dorsally situated respiratory trumpets through which gases are exchanged. The pupal instar is buoyant, in part due to the presence of float hairs on the first abdominal segment, and remains at the surface of the water for the duration of this stage which varies from one to three days.

The adult emerges from the pupal skin (exuvium) and rests either on this skin or on adjacent vegetation before flying off. Soon the adults require to feed. In the case of males the food takes the form of plant juices, in particular the nectar of flowers. Females, however, may feed on plant juices but appear to require blood for the development of their eggs. Exceptions to this do occur, an example being *Aedes communis* which can produce eggs following a diet of sugars alone. In this case additional nutrient requirements have been shown to be obtained from muscle autolysis.

When feeding on blood females take up to about 1·8 times their own weight of fluid, which in absolute terms means that about 1—4 mg of blood is imbibed. The time of day at which females feed on their hosts varies considerably from species to species, but within a given species there is a distinct pattern of biting activity. Thus most *Anopheles* species feed at night while *Haemagogus* species, most *Aedes* species and some *Mansonia* species attack their hosts in the daylight hours (Fig. 18). Quite how the mosquito locates her host is not known, but olfaction, the emission of carbon dioxide from the host, the temperature of the host's body and visual sighting of the host are all known to be important.

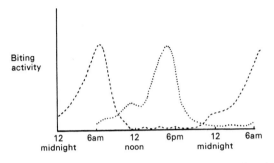

Figure 18 The biting cycles of a diurnal and a nocturnal mosquito. *Anopheles gambiae* — — — — — —, *Aedes aegypti* ··········

Mating usually occurs whilst in flight and in most cases the males form small swarms into which the females fly to copulate. They are attracted to the swarm by the wing-beat noises of the males as well as by their visual and olfactory senses. In many instances females have been known to mate with lone males and in some species, for example *Culex pipiens*, pheromones are secreted by females to attract males.

The longevity of mosquitoes in the wild is not known with certainty but observations suggest that adults of *Anopheles gambiae* live for about nine to eleven days, while those of *Aedes aegypti* survive some five to twenty days. Work on *Anopheles culicifacies* indicates a range of from eight to thirty-four days. The length of life is influenced by both temperature and humidity, for at high temperature and low relative humidity desiccation is rapid. However, under such conditions mosquitoes usually shelter in cool,

humid places like cracks and crevices, inside houses and in burrows
made by other animals. The topic of longevity is an important one
in connection with disease transmission. For instance the malarial
parasites *Plasmodium vivax* and *P. falciparum* take about ten days
to develop in the mosquito at 24°C while at a similar temperature
P. malariae requires twenty-one days and *P. ovale* sixteen days.
Thus the insect must first feed, survive for this length of time and
then feed again in order to transmit the disease and so be a vector
of malaria.

Mosquitoes show a worldwide distribution and the adults are
found in many different types of terrain. Most adults have a limited
flight range of about a kilometre and many seldom stray more than
a few hundred metres unless carried by winds. In addition to the
horizontal distribution of species their vertical distribution also
varies. Thus *Anopheles gambiae* is usually found between 0–10 m
from the ground while *Aedes africanus* normally occupies a zone
some 15–25 m above ground level.

Adults may hibernate and in so doing go through a phase of
complete suspension of activity. In gravid females of some species
aestivation appears to occur in dry seasons and the females emerge
when the rains come and so have suitable habitats in which to
oviposit.

The control of mosquitoes

It is not within the scope of the present text to give a detailed
account of the techniques used to combat mosquitoes, but it is
intended to provide an outline of the methods available for their
control; these are listed below.

1 *By attacking the adult stage*
(a) In endophilic species (i.e. those which enter and rest in
    houses) the walls of rooms can be sprayed with residial
    insecticides such as dichlor-diphenyl-trichlorethane (D D T).
    This has two effects, firstly DDT is toxic to insects and
    secondly it has an irritating effect. The latter point is of

enormous value as the irritant properties persist for a long time and little insecticide has to be used. Thus the method minimizes the danger to other animals and is relatively inexpensive.

Many insects can combat the toxic effects of insecticides by either avoiding treated areas (behavioural effect) or possessing specific enzymes which inactivate the insecticide before it can produce a toxic effect.

(b) It is possible to employ natural virulent parasites of mosquitoes in an attempt to eradicate local populations. Microsporidian protozoans are sometimes the parasites used in such exercises.

(c) The sterile male technique has been utilized with mosquitoes. This involves numerous males being subjected to either gamma radiation or chemosterilants, following which they are released into a population in the wild. The method has been tried with little success with a number of mosquito species including *Aedes aegypti* and *Anopheles quadrimaculatus*.

2 *By attacking the oviposition sites*

(a) Water masses in which mosquitoes breed may be drained, a technique which is economically sound for marshes, etc., can be reclaimed as a result of the disease control measures.

(b) All containers around houses should be kept free of water, which thus removes the breeding sites adjacent to human habitations.

(c) Often the water held by leaves and flowers of plants is used for egg-laying purposes by mosquitoes (e.g. a number of *Mansonia* species) and hence their removal is of considerable value.

(d) It is essential that all domestic and industrial wastes be disposed of efficiently, thus preventing additional breeding sites being established.

(e) Water which is either suspected or known to be used as a breeding site by mosquitoes may be sprayed with either oil or paraffin. This action is of value in combating the larval and pupal stages also.

3 *By attacking the immature stages*

(a) By spraying water masses with either paraffin or oils and so preventing the larvae and pupae from respiring (as suggested above).

(b) By the use of predators of eggs and immatures. For example the fish *Gambusia affinis* has been introduced for this purpose from southern USA. Another fish of use in this respect is *Lebistes reticulatus* (guppy) which can withstand high degrees of organic pollution and is therefore extremely useful in some areas.

Mosquitoes as pests

Mosquitoes transmit a variety of diseases, many to man, some of which will be discussed in a subsequent chapter. However, it must not be forgotten that the mosquito is itself a parasite of man and other animals and may inflict a painful wound and give rise to a condition known as mosquito dermatitis. This happens because the salivary secretion of the mosquito contains proteins foreign to the host and may cause an allergic reaction which lasts from a few hours to several days. In highly susceptible individuals a severe skin reaction may be produced.

The small quantity of blood removed from a host animal by the mosquito is not sufficient to cause an ill effect, even if a large number of bites are received within a short period of time.

3
Sandflies, midges and blackflies

Sandflies

The family Psychodidae is usually divided into two subfamilies, namely the Psychodinae, members of which may cause annoyance by their presence but which are of neither medical nor veterinary importance, and the Phlebotominae, with just one genus, *Phlebotomus*, containing blood-sucking insects which administer extremely painful bites.

Members of the Phlebotominae, commonly known as sandflies, are moth-like, with their bodies and wings covered by small setae (Fig. 19). They are either yellow or light brown in colour and,

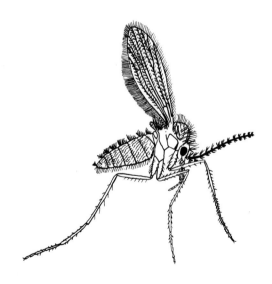

Figure 19 Female *Phlebotomus papatasii*, a sandfly.

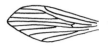

Figure 20 Wing of *Phlebotomus* to show venation.

although small (rarely exceeding 4 mm in length), have relatively long, slender legs. Quite characteristic is the wing shape and venation, with most of the veins running parallel to one another and with few cross veins (Fig. 20), and the long antennae which are made up of sixteen divisions. Sandflies are common in nearly all of the warmer regions of the world.

Although rather short, the mouthparts of sandflies are efficient organs of penetration (Fig. 21). The labrum is broad and tapers to a fine point which carries a number of small spiny projections. Only the female has mandibles, and these take the form of blades which bear numerous small serrations at their tips. The maxillary stylets, which are formed from the galeae, are also blade-like and bear

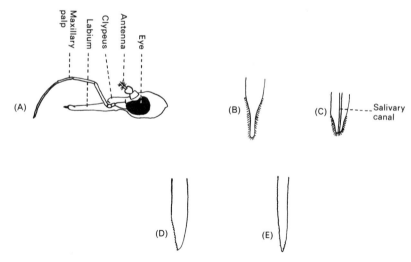

Figure 21 Head and mouthparts of *Phlebotomus* species: A, head and proboscis, lateral view; B, tip of labrum; C, tip of hypopharynx; D, tip of mandible; E, tip of maxillary galea.

numerous fine denticles on their inner margins and a few additional teeth close to their apices on their outer margins. Finally, the labium, which is elongated and channelled to carry the stylets and the hypopharynx, bears a pair of soft labellar lobes distally. The whole of the proboscis is flanked by the paired maxillary palps which are considerably longer than the appendages constituting the proboscis.

As in the mosquitoes, only the maxillary galeae are capable of protraction and retraction, while the mandibles exhibit transverse movements. These are the only two mouthparts used in penetration, and although the labium is flat and blade-like it is not used in piercing but is concerned with the receipt of sensory stimuli. As penetration proceeds the labium is forced up into the membranous posterior wall of the head and so does not enter the wound. When a haemorrhage has been produced blood is sucked up into the gut of the insect by means of a cibarial and a pharyngeal pump. Concomitant with the ingestion of blood is the secretion of saliva. This enters the wound by way of the salivary duct which opens at the tip of the hypopharynx.

Only the female sandfly imbibes blood, the male either feeding on nectar or not feeding at all. Having fed, the females oviposit to produce a few batches of from forty to sixty eggs, these being deposited into the depths of either cracks and crevices (e.g. in brickwork, soil and rubbish) or in animal burrows. The prime requirement of an egg-laying site is apparently that the place should be cool, humid and dark. Quite often the eggs are ejected from the female with considerable force such that they pass to the depths of the holes into which they are laid so ensuring optimal conditions for development.

The eggs hatch in about a week into legless caterpillar-like larvae (Fig. 22) which have greyish-white bodies and dark heads. A number of short setae are distributed over the surface of the body and there are a few characteristically long setae posteriorly. The larvae remain in the place of hatching where they feed on any organic debris which is present. Up to four weeks may elapse before the larva becomes a pale brown pupa which retains the last larval exuvium attached to its posterior end (Fig. 23). After about two weeks in the pupal stage the adult insect emerges.

Adult sandflies are short-lived and are active on warm, still nights, when the females attack animals and man to feed. A few species such as *Phlebotomus papatasii* appear to have a predilection for human blood, but the majority of sandflies are parasites of other animals foremost and attack man incidentally. This is true of, say, *P. argentipes* which feeds on cattle primarily.

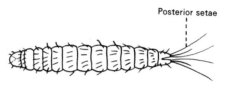

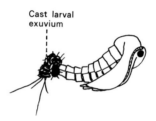

Figure 22 Larva of *Phlebotomus papatasii*.

Figure 23 Pupa of *Phlebotomus papatasii*.

When they bite, the females may cause symptoms due to the development of allergies. These are progressive in that at first the only effect is from the needle-like prick of the proboscis but soon a persistent papule develops which gives both irritation and discomfort.

The control of sandflies relies on a knowledge of their life history and biology. For example it is known that the adults shelter in cool, moist places during the daytime and thus such places are selected for treatment with insecticide sprays. As this type of habitat is also chosen for egg-laying and is the site in which the immature stages are found, it is doubly important that such places should be treated. Adult sandflies are weak fliers, rarely straying more than

50 m, and keep close to the ground. Thus spraying at ground level is to be recommended, including the treatment of ground floors in houses. One great difficulty in sandfly control is a consequence of their small size: they are difficult to bar mechanically for they are able to pass through standard mosquito netting with ease and impunity. Repellent-treated screens are, however, much more effective.

Phlebotomus species are responsible for the transmission of a number of diseases to man, a topic which is dealt with in chapter 9.

Biting midges

These very small, cosmopolitan flies, also commonly called 'no-see-ums' on account of their minuteness, belong to the family Ceratopogonidae. They have a number of characteristic features, among the more important of which are the humped thorax (Fig. 24); the wing venation; the short legs; the long antennae of thirteen divisions which are plumose in the male and pilose in the

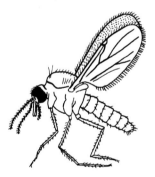

Figure 24 Adult *Culicoides* species.

female; the maxillary palps with five divisions, the third of which is enlarged and equipped with a sensory pit (Fig. 25); and the pattern of the mouthparts. The last feature, however, does not differ radically from that of the blackflies discussed below.

The proboscis of biting midges is short and comprises the usual complement of mouthparts, namely the labium, labrum, mandibles,

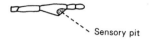

Sensory pit

Figure 25 Maxillary palp of *Culicoides* species.

hypopharynx and maxillary galeae. In the female the mandibles are more strongly developed than in the non-bloodsucking male and are blade-like with a toothed distal region. The left mandible overlies the right (Fig. 26) and the two interlock in a fashion reminiscent of a pair of scissors. However, the mandibles move in a transverse plane only and so do not cut in a scissor-like way as proposed by many authors.

In contrast to the majority of dipteran flies the salivary canal of biting midges traverses the proximal third of the hypopharynx only. After this distance it emerges on to the anterior face of the hypopharynx and continues as an open channel on the surface to the tip of the mouthpart.

Penetration of the host's skin involves movements of the whole proboscis with the exception of the labium which bends backwards

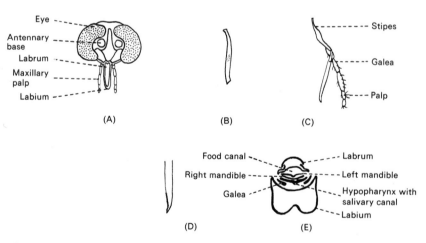

Figure 26 Head and mouthparts of female *Culicoides* species: A, head and proboscis, antennae omitted; B, mandible; C, maxilla; D, tip of galea; E, transverse section through the proboscis.

on the skin surface as the stylets enter. Of the introduced mouth-parts the mandibles and maxillary galeae are responsible for forming the lesion.

After mating each female lays several hundred eggs in shallow waters rich in plants or vegetable matter. These eggs form a gelatinous mass somewhat similar in appearance, although not of course in size, to frog's spawn. The eggs hatch after a few days to give vermiform larvae (Fig. 27) which, like those of the non-biting midges (family Chironomidae), are fully- or semi-aquatic. Chironomid larvae, however, are pigmented with haemoglobin or pigments from ingested food, whereas ceratopogonids are whitish in colour. The biting midge larva has nine abdominal segments, the last of which is equipped with a few characteristic spines and three retractile anal gills which, together with the body cuticle, provide a surface for respiratory exchange. Several weeks or months later the larva becomes a spiny, obtectate pupa (Fig. 28) with two respiratory trumpets, one on each side of the mesothorax. Like the larva it has terminal spines, two in this case, used for anchoring to submerged objects in the water. However, the pupa must breathe gaseous air and rises to the surface at intervals to respire.

One of the more important genera in this family is *Culicoides*, the adults of which measure only 1—3 mm in length. They are obnoxious pests and because of their small size are difficult to keep out of houses and to avoid. The females bite both man and

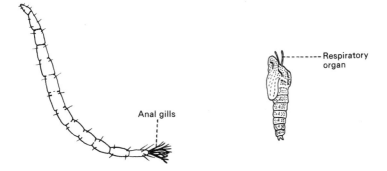

Anal gills

Respiratory organ

Figure 27 Larva of *Culicoides* species.   *Figure 28* Pupa of *Culicoides* species.

D

domesticated animals and give a pricking sensation on biting which is followed by severe irritation. They are most active around dusk and it is at that time that they normally bite. Even so they have been known to attack at other times of the day, especially if disturbed while resting.

As well as causing annoyance *Culicoides* species are known to transmit a number of diseases, including those caused by nematodes of the genera *Dipetalonema*, *Onchocerca* and *Mansonella*. *Culicoides* species have also been named in the spread of a number of virus diseases, such as blue tongue of sheep and horse sickness, and as vectors of the malaria-like organism *Hepatocystis kochi* of monkeys.

The control of biting midges is not easy, in part due to their small size and manoeuvrability. Repellent-treated screens and nets have been usefully employed, as have insecticide emulsions applied to breeding grounds and known habitats.

Blackflies

Like the biting midges the blackflies or buffalo flies, which are grouped in the family Simuliidae, are characterized by their possession of a humped thorax. Once again they are small flies, only 1–5 mm long, with a short proboscis which is powerfully built on similar lines to that of the biting midges.

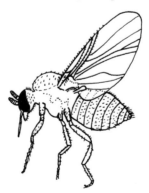

Figure 29 Adult *Simulium* species.

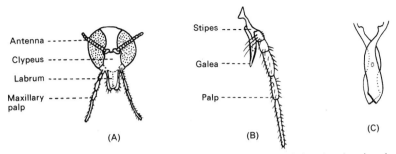

Figure 30 Head and mouthparts of female *Simulium* species: A, head and proboscis, anterior view; B, maxilla; C, mandibles in interlocked position.

Despite the similarities between ceratopogonids and simuliids it is possible to separate them using a number of criteria. First, most buffalo flies are black in colour; hence their other common name. However, care must be exercised here, for exceptions occur with some species being brown or even yellow. A number of absolute characters will nevertheless serve to distinguish them with ease. Thus in simuliids the antennae are composed of only eleven divisions and are neither plumose nor pilose. Also, the wings are always broad and have a venation which is quite unmistakable (Fig. 29).

With regard to the mouthparts (Fig. 30) the stylets are weaker in the male than in the female, with the latter being the only haematophagous sex. As in the ceratopogonids the mandibles have the appearance of scissors with the left blade lying above the right, but again they move transversely only. The maxillary blades are the galeae, and each is equipped with a number of teeth. There are also a pair of maxillary stipites located basally and two long five-jointed palps. The labium is wide and soft and is hollowed to house the maxillary galeae, the broad flattened hypopharynx and the mandibles. The labrum is also broad and is equipped with denticles distally and has a hollowed lower surface.

In common with the biting midges the salivary canal does not extend the full length of the hypopharynx as a closed tube. It opens to the surface in the proximal half and runs to the tip of the hypopharynx as a groove.

Penetration of the host is brought about by a cutting action of the mandibles followed by insertion of the galeae which enlarge the wound. In contrast to the biting midges which have well-developed cibarial and pharyngeal pumps blackflies draw fluids into their alimentary tracts mainly by means of a powerful cibarial pump, the pharyngeal apparatus being poorly developed.

Batches of several hundred eggs are laid by females on stones and plants just below the surface of rapidly flowing waters, the female either completely submerging herself to lay or depositing eggs on leaves which then sink under the weight of the eggs. In some cases the female has been observed to lay her eggs just above the water level such that they are submerged with the movement of the water. This is not a true equivalent of the flood-water method employed by *Aedes* mosquitoes, as the eggs of simuliids cannot withstand appreciable desiccation.

The eggs hatch after a few days to a couple of weeks to give cylindrical larvae (Fig. 31 A). They maintain their hold on the egg case by means of a silken thread secreted by the salivary glands until able to attach to a more substantial submerged object using a circlet of small hooklets on the last body segment. Anteriorly, on the ventral surface of the first thoracic segment, there is a short proleg which is also armed with a circlet of hooks. These holdfasts are used by the larva in locomotion, the insect attaching by them alternatively and looping along. It is perhaps worth mentioning that another method of locomotion may be employed in which the larva anchors itself to a point on the substratum by means of a

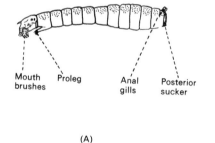
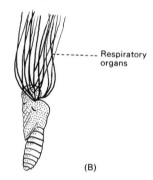

Mouth   Proleg   Anal   Posterior
brushes   gills   sucker

Respiratory
organs

(A)

(B)

Figure 31 Simulium species: A, larva; B, pupa.

thread, releases its hold with the hooklets and then drifts
downstream. The larvae feed by means of a pair of mouthbrushes
or fans which produce a feeding current so bringing suspended
particles into the mouth. Occasionally larger particles of food may
be taken and there are reports of larvae feeding on pieces of algae
and on small animals.

A total of six moults occur in a life cycle before the pupal instar
is reached. Using silk from the salivary glands the last larval stage
spins a cocoon in which pupation takes place, the cocoon being
securely attached to a stone or something similar in the stream.
The immobile pupa (Fig. 31 B) is obtectate and respires by means
of a pair of arborescent respiratory tubes, the branches of which
emerge from the cocoon. Within three to fourteen days the imaginal
insect is ready to appear and is carried to the surface on an air
bubble which has accumulated on the inside of the pupal skin.

Blackflies are virtually ubiquitous, being found from the poles to
the tropics in such places where running waters exist. The flies are
a particular problem in warmer lands, especially when they attack in
swarms, for not only do they cause severe annoyance and pain
when they bite, but the lesions are often troublesome and develop
into vesicles and papules. Adult flies are diurnal and are especially
active in the morning and evening, although they are often to be
seen in the heat of the day in the brightest of sunlight.

Many authorities recognize several closely related genera of blackflies, with the better-known members being placed in the genus
Simulium. Among the important species are *S. columbaczense*
from the shores of the Danube, *S. venustum* of North America
which transmits the protozoan, *Leucocytozoon*, and *S. damnosum*
of Africa which infects man with the notorious nematode
Onchocerca volvulus.

Control measures against *Simulium* species are again difficult,
the flies being able to pass through standard netting and having a
flight range of some 15 km or more. As with other species nets and
clothing treated with repellents are of some value, as is also the
controlled addition of insecticides to rivers to kill the immature
stages.

4

Tsetse flies and other Muscidae

The tsetse flies are placed in the genus *Glossina*, all members of which are confined to the mainland of Africa south of the Tropic of Cancer and to some of the outlying islands including Zanzibar but not Malagasy. There is, in addition, a record of *G. tachinoides* from southern Arabia.

Although some authors place the tsetse flies in the family Glossinidae of the suborder Cyclorrhapha, most would agree that they are closely related to the muscid flies and therefore classify them in the family Muscidae. Tsetse flies are large but narrow-bodied flies (Fig. 32) and vary in colour from yellow to dark brown. They may be identified by their characteristic forwardly directed proboscis, their antennae and their wing venation. It is not easy to separate males from females but it is useful to know that females are invariably larger than males. Identification may be made with certainty, however, by inspection of the external genitalia.

The tsetse wing venation (Fig. 33) is characteristic and is of value in providing supplementary means of identification. The

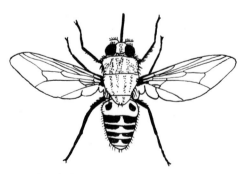

Figure 32 Adult tsetse, dorsal view.

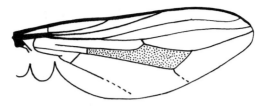

Figure 33 Wing venation of tsetse. The characteristic 'hatchet' cell is stippled.

homologies of the veins have not as yet been determined and they are best numbered rather than named. The space or cell located between the fourth and fifth longitudinal veins has the shape of a hatchet or cleaver and is unlike that found in members of any other genus.

The head of the tsetse bears two large compound eyes as well as three simple eyes, or ocelli. From it arise the mouthparts which will be discussed later and the characteristic antennae which are composed of three divisions, or podomeres, the two more proximal of which are much smaller than the distal one. From the base of the distal podomere there arises a structure known as the arista which bears a single row of between seventeen and twenty-nine branched setae along its anterior edge (Fig. 34). The antennae are sensitive to many stimuli, especially odours, humidity and temperature.

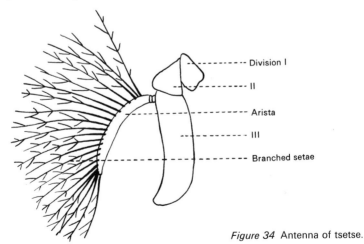

Figure 34 Antenna of tsetse.

Although it is difficult to distinguish between the twenty-two species of tsetses using morphological criteria, they fall into three apparently natural groups with regard to their ecological requirements. These groupings, which are of uncertain taxonomic status, are the *fusca* group, the *palpalis* group and the *morsitans* group. Of the three the *fusca* group is thought to be the most primitive and because of their preference for forest areas most of the species have little or no contact with man. This group has a very wide distribution which coincides approximately with the combined distributions of the *palpalis* and *morsitans* groups. The areas in which tsetses occur are commonly known as 'fly belts'.

In general, the distribution of members of the *palpalis* group coincides with the presence of rain forests. Actually, members of this group have extended their range by following the courses of rivers through other types of territory and thus in some cases have a strip-like geographical occurrence. Because of the presence of human habitations in the vicinity of waterways, owing to their value in transportation, man has come into close contact with species in this group and hence these insects rate as important vectors of human disease.

The species which constitute the *morsitans* group are, in general, found in dry regions, being common in open savannah and absent in the extensive rain forests of West Africa. Once again, because of the presence of man in open grassland areas adjacent to woodlands for purposes of agriculture and the tending of stock, *morsitans* group tsetses are common human parasites.

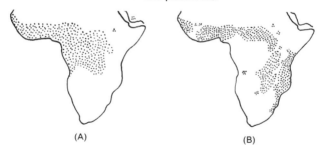

(A)   (B)

Figure 35 The distribution of A, the *palpalis* group and B, the *morsitans* group compiled from available records.

The areas in which members of the *morsitans* and *palpalis* groups of flies are found are shown in Fig. 35, and the relationship between their breeding—resting and feeding areas is shown in Fig. 36. As can be seen from the diagram the tsetses need the juxtaposition of two quite distinct types of environment to act as their breeding—resting ground and their feeding ground. In some instances three different terrains are required, with the flies utilizing separate habitats for breeding and resting. Tsetses are therefore not found in localities with uniform features, as, for example, uninterrupted tropical rain forests and large expanses of open savannah.

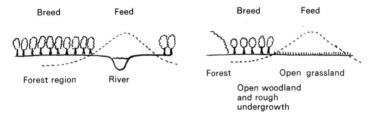

Figure 36 Diagrammatic representation of the relationship between the breeding and feeding grounds of A, the *palpalis* group and B, the *morsitans* group. Superimposed upon each is a graph of biting activity.

Mouthparts and feeding

The tsetse proboscis is composed of a labium, labrum and hypopharynx. When the insect is not feeding the proboscis is enclosed by the paired inwardly grooved maxillary palps (Fig. 37). The labium is longer than the labrum and the labella at its tip are modified to form an organ of penetration and are not the soft, suctorial bodies found in most muscid flies. A hollow in the labrum forms the food canal and this is completed below by the labium, the two structures being held together by means of a number of interlocking ridges. Also contained in this canal is the long, slender hypopharynx which, as in many other insects, is a forward extension of the common salivary duct (Fig. 40).

The labium consists of two plates, the ventral theca and the

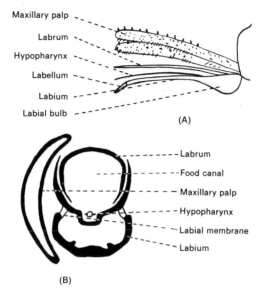

Figure 37 Mouthparts of tsetse: A, lateral view with stylets separated; B, transverse section through the proboscis (the maxillary palp is shown on one side only).

dorsal labial gutter (Fig. 37), which run the length of the mouth-part, being joined together laterally by flexible membranes. The gutter is fixed to the labrum by the interlocking ridges, but the theca, which is continuous with the labella, can move and as it is pulled backwards by muscles housed in the labial bulb it everts the labella by some 45–65 μm and so exposes the teeth and rasps (Fig. 39). The labella are retracted by the contraction of other muscles in the labial bulb which have long tendons running to the lobes.

Insertion of the proboscis into the skin of a host results from the

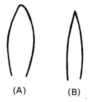

Figure 38 Tips of A, labrum and B, hypopharynx of tsetse.

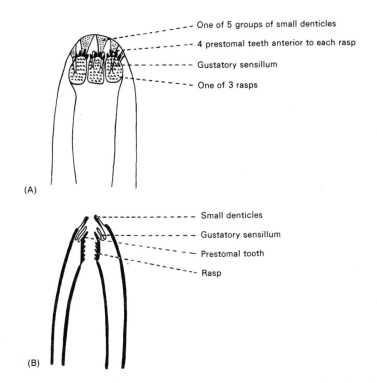

One of 5 groups of small denticles

4 prestomal teeth anterior to each rasp

Gustatory sensillum

One of 3 rasps

(A)

Small denticles

Gustatory sensillum

Prestomal tooth

Rasp

(B)

Figure 39 Labellum of tsetse fly from inside (A) and a longitudinal section through the labella (B).

rapid inversion and eversion of the armed labella, augmented by downward thrusts of the head. Once the surface layer (stratum corneum) of the skin has been pierced the flexible proboscis is moved backwards and forwards until a large blood capillary is located and punctured. This indeed explains the variation which occurs in the length of time required by the flies to complete engorgement (from one to ten minutes), for the penetration of a blood vessel is purely a matter of chance and several attempts at probing may be necessary. Throughout the engorgement period saliva is ejected intermittently by the action of the salivary pump and some is reimbibed, so preventing the ingested blood from clotting in the mouthparts and the alimentary canal.

The liquid food is drawn up through the food canal by means of the cibarial pump, which is equipped with large external dilator muscles but which returns to its original shape by its own elasticity. At the posterior end of the pump there is a sphincter muscle to control the movement of fluids into the gut and prevent regurgitation. The cibarium leads directly to the oesophagus, there apparently being no pharynx, and the blood meal is conveyed to the proventriculus and the crop (Fig. 40). Only when the tsetse is nearing full engorgement does the blood pass to the midgut region. The whole of the mesenteron is lined by a chitinous layer, the peritrophic membrane, secreted by the proventriculus, which is permeable to digestive juices and products of digestion. The membrane is secreted throughout the life of the fly and is eroded away at its posterior end which extends into the hindgut. The

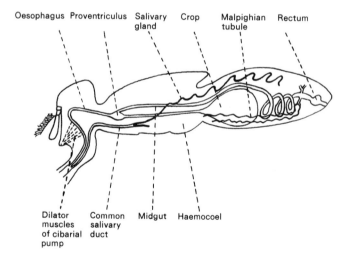

Figure 40 Longitudinal section of a tsetse showing features of the alimentary canal.

rectum of the hindgut is equipped with glands to withdraw water from the faeces if the fly is becoming dehydrated.

At about the time of engorgement and continuing for some thirty minutes after the withdrawal of the mouthparts a clear fluid which originates from the recently imbibed blood is excreted from the anus. This 'primary excretion' consists of water and salts and presumably is a means of providing the fly with room for more food as well as removing excess water and hence weight prior to taking off from the host. Despite this measure the tsetse cannot fly efficiently immediately after a meal and makes for nearby tree cover, where it rests on the underside of a branch. Here it continues to excrete excess water and salts once more, this period being called the phase of 'secondary excretion'.

Both male and female tsetses feed exclusively on the blood of reptiles, birds and mammals, and they neither feed on plant juices nor possess the necessary amylases to digest such food. Some of the midgut cells of these flies contain bacteroids which are thought to be symbiotic and of value to the fly in supplying vitamins not otherwise available to a wholly haematophagous animal.

Life history
Tsetse flies are unusual, although not unique amongst insects, in that they are larviparous. The eggs pass into the uterus singly and hatch at this site, the pharate larva breaking through the egg membranes with the aid of its 'egg tooth'. Once the membranes have ruptured they are pulled away from the larva by means of a special organ on the floor of the uterus called the choriothete. The first-stage larva remains in the uterus and is nourished by the secretion from the uterine, vitelline or 'milk glands' as they are varyingly called (Fig. 41). Although the mouth of the larva lies close to the common opening of these glands, the secretion is in fact passed into the uterus and is not sucked directly from the duct of the gland (Fig. 42). When the first-stage larva moults the choriothete removes its exuvium, but then it degenerates and does not aid the moult from the second- to the third-stage larva, this

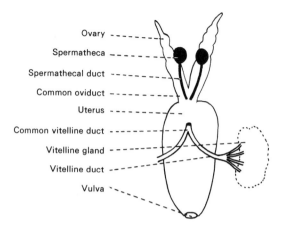

Figure 41 Reproductive system of a female tsetse.

skin being removed as the larva is passed through the vaginal opening at parturition. However, the choriothete then redevelops to be fully functional in time for the next larva to develop in the uterus.

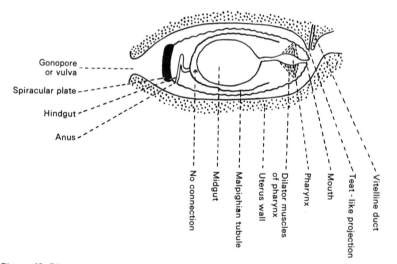

Figure 42 Diagrammatic longitudinal section of the uterus of a tsetse showing a larva *in situ*.

While in the latter stages of life within the uterus and after its liberation from the female, the larva breathes by means of a tracheal system and associated stigmal plates which are pierced by about five hundred small spiracular openings. When inside the female the larva is orientated such that the posterior respiratory plates are located close to the female gonopore and hence are functional even though the larva is in an enclosed space (Fig. 42).

As indicated above, it is the third-stage larva which is extruded from the female; this is deposited on to soft soil in shady places. It is apodous and its most obvious feature is the paired posterior respiratory lobes, which are black in colour. At the anterior end of the larva are two black rod-like structures known as the antenno-maxillary organs which are thought to be sensory in function. The free-living larva does not feed and in fact its alimentary tract is incomplete in that the midgut and hindgut are not joined (Fig. 42). The gut is made functional in the fourth-stage larva, when excreta is voided for the first time.

The third-stage larva is motile for about an hour only, and burrows rapidly into the soil to a depth of a few centimetres. It soon becomes immobile and its cuticle hardens and darkens in colour. This is the puparium (Fig. 43), a stage generally found in the Cyclorrhapha. Inside the puparial integument the larva undergoes yet another moult to become a fourth-stage larva and then moults a further time to become a true pupa, still encased by the puparial cuticle of the third larval stage. Eventually the adult is formed from the pupa and escapes from the puparium aided by an eversible membranous sac contained within the head called the ptilinum and found in all members of the Cyclorrhapha. This same structure may also be of considerable use in helping the newly emerged adult to escape from the soil in which it is buried. Once the cuticle of the fly has hardened the ptilinum is no longer eversible but its position is indicated by the ptilinal suture. The total time taken from the time of puparium formation to the emergence of the adult varies from twenty to ninety days depending on the ambient temperature.

The adult females are capable of mating almost immediately

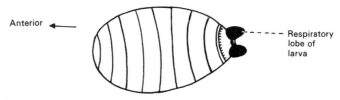

Anterior ← — — — Respiratory lobe of larva

Figure 43 Puparium of tsetse.

after emergence, but males can mate only after four to seven days from the time of emergence. Females require to mate just once in a lifetime and it is probable that one mating is normal, the spermatozoa from the male being stored in a pair of seminal receptacles or spermathecae. It is not known with certainty which sex is attracted to which, but swarms of males are often seen and it is likely that females are attracted into these, as is the case with mosquitoes. However, as with mosquitoes, lone males and females will also mate. Copulation whilst in flight appears to be normal but it may take place on the ground equally successfully.

Female tsetses have a pair of ovaries which produce eggs alternately, the eggs passing to the uterus by way of the oviducts for further development. Although doubtless subject to enormous variation it appears that an average of six larvae are produced by each female, with only a single larva developing at any one time. About ten days pass from the hatching of the egg to the emergence of the third-stage larva from the female gonopore.

Unfed tsetses fly very fast and remain close to the ground. They hunt mainly by sight and take a blood meal, on average, every three to five days. The feed may last from one to ten minutes and during this time some 60 mg of blood are imbibed. Having fed, the tsetses are very heavy, even after excreting fluid prior to leaving the host (see above). As they therefore have difficulty taking off and gaining height, they make for nearby cover to rest for a half an hour or so. During this time they remove most of the water from the blood meal, thus allowing them to fly efficiently once more.

Because of the need to seek refuge immediately after engorgement tsetses feed close to trees, and usually in their shade. The flies are quite discriminate in their choice of hosts and thus a species of mammal may abound in an area and yet not be used as a food source whereas less numerous animals may be parasitized almost exclusively. The reason for the choice of host is unknown, but it is not due to the nutritional value of the blood, which is almost identical in all mammals. As an example of the discrimination of hosts *Glossina morsitans* may be cited, which feeds mainly on suids and bovids and to a lesser extent on birds and other mammals including man. A few tsetses, namely the subspecies of *G. palpalis*, appear to be less discriminate in their choice of hosts.

Nearly all tsetse species bite during the daytime. In *G. pallidipes* the males tend to bite mostly in the afternoon and show a peak at 1500–1600 hours, whilst the females exhibit a peak in biting activity from late morning to late afternoon (1100–1700 hours). In contrast to this *G. longipennis* usually attacks just before sunset and at dawn and shows little signs of activity during the day, whilst *G. brevipalpis* is exceptional in that it is nocturnal, feeding mainly on moonlit nights.

Varying estimates have been made with regard to the longevity of adult tsetses in the wild. It would appear that the length of life depends on the season and environmental conditions, such that females live from six to fifteen weeks and males from four to eight weeks.

Control of tsetse flies

Control measures have been attempted against all accessible stages of *Glossina* with varying success. Eggs are not laid and the larvae are, of course, difficult to combat due to the short free-living phase of the instar. Similarly, the pupae, because of their subterranean existence, present an equally troublesome problem. However, techniques aimed at controlling pupae have been implemented, the more common employing insecticides, hyperparasites of the instar and mechanical methods. Most of the effort in tsetse control has been directed against the adult stage. Traps of various types and adhesive surfaces have been tried with only marginal effects, but modification of the terrain, destruction of game and the use of insecticides have given much more promising results.

The clearing of bushes and thickets, particularly those surrounding human habitation and close to roads, by burning or by chemical or mechanical means gives an important method of controlling adults of species which require shade and shelter (e.g. *G. palpalis* and the pupae of many species of tsetse). The method is, however, of less value in combatting many open parkland species like *G. morsitans*.

Attempts have been made to kill off game animals in some regions and so remove the common food source of tsetses. Indeed, the elimination of antelopes from Rhodesia has successfully controlled *G. morsitans* but in Botswana their removal had little effect because other animals were also used as hosts. This underlines the importance of a sound knowledge of the biology of insects before such methods of control are attempted. It must also be added that such control techniques are rather drastic in that many thousands of animals are required to be slaughtered.

Finally, we come to the use of insecticides to control the flies. These have been used directly on animals, particularly cattle, in which case they either kill the flies or discourage them from biting, as well as being sprayed from the air over large areas. The most common agents used have been DDT and benzene hexachloride or hexachlorocyclohexane (BHC), and they have been responsible for drastic reductions in the number of flies in localized areas. There are, of course, objections to mass spraying as the chemicals used are biocides and not simply insecticides; even so the substances

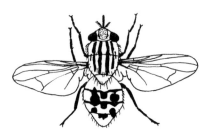

Figure 44 Adult *Stomoxys*.

often fail to reach pupae and adult flies in densely foliated places. Coating animals with insecticides is of considerable value but, unfortunately, the toxicity of the insecticides soon wears off, although as mentioned elsewhere the irritant qualities of the chemicals may persist for longer periods.

Stomoxys

In common with *Glossina* this genus comprises biting species, the best known of which is the ubiquitous *Stomoxys calcitrans*, commonly known as the stable fly or biting house fly (Fig. 44). Male and female flies attack a wide range of hosts including horses, sheep, cattle and man, lacerating the skin tissues with mouthparts of similar design to those of tsetse flies (Fig. 45). In fact, stable flies share many features in common with tsetses but may be

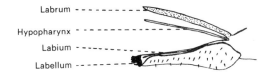

Figure 45 Mouthparts of *Stomoxys*, lateral view.

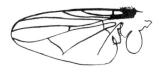

Figure 46 Wing venation of *Stomoxys calcitrans*.

differentiated from them by the form of the arista, which in *Stomoxys* has unbranched setae on the dorsal surface only; the wing venation (Fig. 46); the extremely small maxillary palps; and the patterning of the thorax and abdomen. The dorsal surface of the thorax of *S. calcitrans* is grey but has four longitudinal dark stripes, the lateral ones terminating short of the posterior margin of the scutellum. The abdomen also has a grey background but has three dark patches on the second and third segments.

The female fly lays her eggs either in faeces or organic matter, and has a notable predilection for animal bedding which has been moistened with urine or contaminated with faeces. Batches of about twenty-five to fifty eggs are laid and each female is capable of producing in the region of 750 eggs in the course of her lifetime. The eggs hatch one to seven days later, and the emergent maggot-like larvae feed on the vegetation and become fully mature in two to four weeks. Larvae of *Stomoxys* may be positively identified by the design of their posterior spiracular plates (Fig. 47). Once

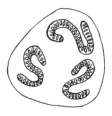

Figure 47 Spiracular plate of the larva of *Stomoxys*.

mature, the larval skin darkens and hardens to become a puparial case inside which the pupa forms. Some five to ten days are required for pupation and the emergent females must feed prior to oviposition.

Adult stable flies have the habit of interrupting their feeding and recommencing either at another site on the same host or quite commonly on another host. This habit permits the mechanical carriage of blood parasites from one animal to another and helps to explain the importance of *Stomoxys* as a disease-transmitter.

Lyperosia

Members of this genus are small, haematophagous flies with a single metallic grey stripe down an otherwise dark thorax. The wing venation (Fig. 48) and arista are essentially similar to those of *Stomoxys* but the maxillary palps are about the same length as the proboscis (Fig. 49). An important species in this genus is *Lyperosia irritans* (horn fly), found in many European countries, which sucks blood from cattle and subsequently lays its eggs in their newly deposited faeces. The eggs hatch in a day or so and the larvae burrow into the dung and feed on its contents. Some four days after hatching the larvae become puparia and about a week later the adults emerge.

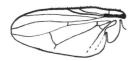

Figure 48 Wing venation of *Lyperosia irritans.*

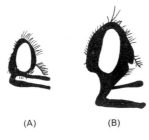

(A)   (B)

Figure 49 Outlines of the heads of A, *Lyperosia* and B, *Haematobia.*

Haematobia

Species contained within this genus have an almost identical life cycle to those of *Lyperosia* outlined above. However, they differ morphologically and the adults of *Haematobia* species may be recognized by their aristae which have setae on both dorsal and ventral margins; their clubbed maxillary palps which are slightly shorter than the proboscis (Fig. 49); and their wing venation (Fig. 50).

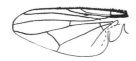

Figure 50 Wing venation of *Haematobia stimulans.*

Two important species deserve mention: *H. stimulans* from Europe, and *H. irritans* from North America, which with *Lyperosia irritans* shares the common name of horn fly. The latter *Haematobia* species is found around the base of the horns and the backs of cattle, and occasionally horses and sheep. The flies remain in close contact with their hosts and leave them only when either flying to another host or depositing their eggs in the animal's faeces. Adult flies are persistent biters and, as they occur in swarms, give rise to extensive skin lesions which commonly become secondarily infected.

Musca

This genus and the next two to be considered contain members which differ from the previous muscids mentioned in that they are non-biting flies. Nevertheless, they are extremely important because of their habit of visiting both faeces and food and so carrying disease organisms to animals. Some non-biting Muscidae are also important as they act as intermediate hosts for a number of important parasites (see below).

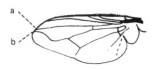

Figure 51 Wing venation of *Musca domestica.*

Figure 52 Antenna of *Musca domestica.*

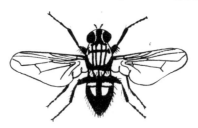

Figure 53 Adult *Musca domestica.*

Musca domestica is the cosmopolitan common house fly and may be recognized by the wing venation, in particular the sharp forward bend of the fourth longitudinal vein (Fig. 51); the arista with its double row of unbranched setae (Fig. 52); and the coloration of the thorax, which is grey dorsally with four bold longitudinal stripes, and the abdomen, which is pale but with a median dark stripe and a broad, dark posterior border (Fig. 53). The mouthparts are adapted for imbibing liquid and soluble foods, the latter being liquefied with either exuded salivary secretion or regurgitated crop fluids.

Females lay batches of from 100 to 150 eggs and produce a total of about 600 during their lifetime. These are oviposited in manure, refuse or other organic matter and normally hatch within twenty-four hours. The larva (Fig. 54 A) moults three times before becoming a pupal instar and, as with many other muscids, the third-stage larva buries itself in the ground, after which its cuticle becomes the puparial casing. The larval stage lasts for between four and seven days, while the duration of the pupal instar is from three to twenty-five days, the times being modified by the ambient temperature.

The maggots may be identified by their posterior spiracular plates (Fig. 54 C) whilst the puparium (Fig. 54 B) is

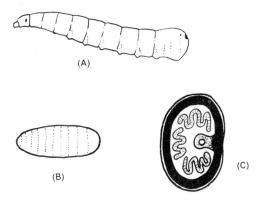

(A)

(B)   (C)

Figure 54 Musca domestica: A, larva; B, puparium; C, posterior spiracular plate of larva.

characteristically ovoid and dark in colour. As the larvae often live and feed in faeces they may ingest the eggs of parasites and pathogenic bacteria voided from the host animal. Indeed *M. domestica* is the proven intermediate host of the nematodes *Setaria labiopapillosa* of bovines and *Habronema microstoma* and *H. megastoma* of equines. Although bacteria may be ingested by larvae and persist to the adult stage it is more common for such disease organisms to be taken up directly by the adult when visiting faeces either to feed or oviposit. Such organisms may either be taken directly into the alimentary canal or simply adhere to the bodies of flies. If the flies then visit human food substances some of the pathogens on their body surfaces may be transferred directly on to the food, while in an attempt to liquefy the food for their own requirements crop secretions and hence imbibed organisms are expelled to be later ingested by a host animal.

Muscina

Members of this genus, for example *Muscina stabulans*, the cosmopolitan non-biting house fly, have life stages and a life cycle which are extremely similar to those of *Musca*. However, diagnosis may be made on the basis of the wing venation of the adult (Fig. 55) and the posterior spiracular plates of the larva. As with *Musca*, this genus is noteworthy for its mechanical dissemination of pathogens from faecal materials.

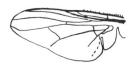

Figure 55 Wing venation of *Muscina stabulans*.

Fannia

Two important species of this fly requiring mention are *Fannia canicularis*, the lesser house fly, and *F. scalaris*, the latrine fly.

    F. canicularis is dark grey in colour with three darker stripes on the dorsum of the thorax. It may additionally be identified by the absence of setae on the arista and by its wing venation (Fig. 56). The larvae of this genus breed in decaying organic materials and are easily recognized by their dorso-ventrally flattened bodies from

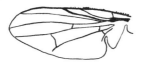

Figure 56 Wing venation of *Fannia canicularis*.

which project numerous lateral processes (Fig. 57 A, B). As far as shape is concerned, the puparium resembles the larva but it is dark in colour with a rigid tegument. *F. scalaris* is similar to *F. canicularis* in most essential detail except that it breeds in human faeces and that the projections from the larva are more complex (Fig. 57 C).

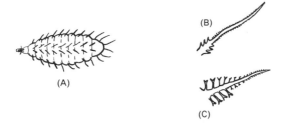

Figure 57 Fannia species : A, third-stage larva of *Fannia canicularis* with details of the projections (B) ; C, details of a projection from *Fannia scalaris*.

5

Blowflies, keds and horseflies

Blowflies

Most people are familiar with the large buzzing bluebottles and
their allies, but usually think of them not as disease-producing
organisms but as mere nuisances. However, from a parasitological
standpoint, members of the cyclorrhaphan family Calliphoridae are
important on two counts: first because, like various muscid flies,
they may visit human faeces and subsequently alight on human
foods, so contaminating them, and second the larvae of several
species may parasitize wounds and lesions of man and other
animals. Some species of Calliphoridae, for example those of the
genus *Calliphora*, may lay their eggs in decomposing animal matter,
meat and fish destined for human consumption, or even dirty
wounds and lesions on the body surface of various animals. Thus
their larvae may occasionally be parasitic and are said to exhibit
facultative myiasis. On the other hand, members of genera such as
Callitroga and *Chrysomyia*, the screw-worm flies, always lay their
eggs on living flesh and have abandoned the non-parasitic habits of
Calliphora. These are said to show obligate myiasis.

There are a large number of genera of Calliphoridae, and only
the parasitologically important ones are listed below together with a
few details of their structure and biology.

Calliphora

These are the well-known bluebottle flies of which there are
numerous species found throughout the world. In general they are
dull blue in colour and range from 8 to 14 mm in length. One of the
more common species is *Calliphora erythrocephala*, a large robust
fly which may be identified by its wing venation (Fig. 58) and the

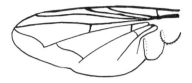

Figure 58 Wing of *Calliphora erythrocephala.*

red coloration of the eyes and parts of the head (the genae). A second species of importance which is similar morphologically but which has black genae is *C. vomitoria*. The larvae of these species are normally found in meat which has not been adequately covered, so permitting its use as an oviposition site, although as indicated above they may also occur in unclean wounds and rotting organic matter. The white, wedge-shaped larvae (maggots) may be identified by means of their posterior spiracular plates (Fig. 59).

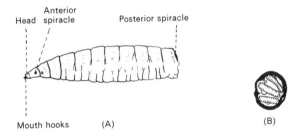

Figure 59 Calliphora erythrocephala: A, larva; B, larval spiracular plate.

Lucilia
Members of this genus are responsible for the condition known as 'blowfly strike' of sheep in a number of countries including South Africa and Australia, where the species responsible is *Lucilia cuprina*, and in most temperate lands such as Britain, where *L. sericata* is the offending insect. The adult flies are metallic green in colour and therefore known as greenbottles. They range in length from 9 to 15 mm. The female lays her eggs in the wounds, carcasses and soiled wool of sheep in particular and the larvae hatch within a few days, feed on the tissues and their exudates

and moult twice to become third-stage larvae, the spiracular plates of which are shown in Fig. 60. When mature these normally leave the host to pupate in the ground, although on occasions they may undergo pupation in the fleece.

Most commonly the adult flies select wool soiled with urine, faeces or blood. Control of the flies thus entails emphasis on hygiene as well as the external administration of various insecticide compounds such as dieldrin and BHC.

Figure 60 Spiracular plate of *Lucilia sericata* larva.

Figure 61 Spiracular plate of *Phormia regina* larva.

Phormia

Like *Lucilia* members of this genus also cause 'strike' in sheep. The adults resemble small bluebottles but have a purple-black thorax with a metallic sheen and a bluish-black abdomen. They are about 10 mm in length. The larvae are basically similar to those of other members of the family but may be identified by the appearance of their posterior spiracular plates (Fig. 61).

Phormia is a genus restricted to the north temperate region, an important example of which is *P. terraenovae* found in Britain.

Chrysomyia

The Old World screw-worm fly, *Chrysomyia bezziana*, of Africa, southern Asia and parts of the Far East attacks sheep and, less often, other animals including man. This species shows a predilection for wounds and abscesses in man, but the female will also lay her egg batches in body orifices like the ear, nose and urino-genital passages.

Adult flies are metallic blue-green in colour and the third-stage

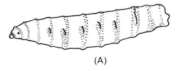

(A)   (B)

Figure 62 Chrysomyia bezziana : A, larva ; B, spiracular plate of larva.

larvae (Fig. 62 A) are cream and covered with numerous short, black spines arranged as circlets on the anterior part of each segment. Larvae of *Chrysomyia* species may also be identified by means of their posterior spiracular plates (Fig. 62 B).

Callitroga

The adults of this genus are also referred to as screw-worm flies, one of the more notorious being *Callitroga hominivorax* of North and South America. The female fly lays large batches of eggs close to wounds and sores on humans, cattle, pigs and equines, and the larvae hatch in a few hours, penetrate into the skin tissues by way of the lesion, feed, and mature in less than a week. At this stage they are about 15 mm long, with bands of spines on most of their body segments and characteristic posterior spiracular plates (Fig. 63). They then leave the host and pupate on the ground, and in about three days give rise to adult flies.

Figure 63 Spiracular plate of *Callitroga hominivorax* larva.

Cordylobia

Cordylobia anthropophaga, the 'tumbu fly' of Africa, is an important insect, for its larvae commonly parasitize man and dogs. The broadly built adult is less than 12 mm long, and is light brown in colour with two darker patches on the thorax and a dark patch on the posterior abdominal segments. Females oviposit in the bedding of animals including man and the larvae hatch in a few days and burrow into the skin almost anywhere on the body. One or two weeks later the larvae are mature and lie within a swelling on the body surface. They are about 12 mm long and their cuticle is covered by small spines (Fig. 64). After leaving the host three to four weeks are required before pupation is completed.

Sarcophaga

This is a cosmopolitan genus and the females are viviparous, depositing their larvae into unclean wounds, ulcers and natural

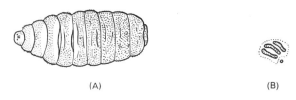

(A)   (B)

Figure 64 Cordylobia anthropophaga: A, larva; B, spiracular plate of larva.

orifices of man and sometimes other animals. Although body
lesions are the main egg-laying sites, decaying organic debris may
also be selected by females. *Sarcophaga haemorrhoidalis*, which
occurs in Europe, Africa, Asia and America, is a large fly, and is
grey in colour with longitudinal black stripes on the dorsal region
of the thorax and scattered dark patches on the abdomen. The
larvae are similar to those of *Calliphora* although the spiracular
plates are of a different design (Fig. 65).

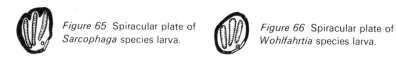

Figure 65 Spiracular plate of
Sarcophaga species larva.

Figure 66 Spiracular plate of
Wohlfahrtia species larva.

Wohlfahrtia

Species of *Wohlfahrtia* are, in common with those of *Sarcophaga*,
viviparous and have similar adults, although those of the former
have a spotted abdominal design. *Wohlfahrtia magnifica*, the 'Old
World flesh fly', is found throughout the Mediterranean region, the
Middle East and the USSR. The larvae are deposited into body
openings, usually the ear, of man and other animals such as sheep.
Larvae may be identified by means of their spiracular plates
(Fig. 66).

Booponus

Booponus intonsus, the 'foot maggot fly' of cattle and other
animals, is found in the Philippines and in Celebes and is a
yellowish-brown fly of similar size to *Musca domestica*. The female
lays her eggs attached to hairs on the bodies of cattle and the

larvae hatch and penetrate into the skin to produce lesions from which the posterior ends of the larvae protrude. In two to three weeks the larvae mature and drop from the host to pupate in the ground. One or two weeks are then required for the development of the adult instar.

Auchmeromyia

The best-known member of this genus is *Auchmeromyia luteola*, commonly called the 'Congo floor maggot fly'. Adult flies may be recognized by their yellowish-brown bodies which have a number of dark longitudinal stripes on the thorax and a dark posterior abdominal region. The second abdominal segment is quite characteristic, being elongated and accounting for about half the length of the abdomen. The larvae (Fig. 67) do not stay on their host all of the time but remain in cracks and crevices by day and emerge at night to feed on human and other hosts by piercing their skin and extracting tissue fluids.

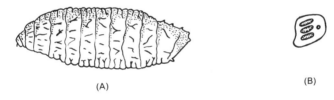

(A)   (B)

Figure 67 Auchmeromyia luteola: A, larva; B, spiracular plate of larva.

Keds

The keds and their allies are classed in another of the cyclorrhaphan families, the Hippoboscidae. Both males and females feed on the blood of either birds or mammals and show considerable adaptation to an ectoparasitic mode of life. Thus the head and body are flattened dorso-ventrally, there is a tendency in the group to lose the wings and the legs bear strong recurved claws. The antennae are composed of a single joint only and may be found in a depression in the relatively small head in some species such as *Melophagus ovinus*. Females of this family are larviparous and, like tsetse flies, the larvae are ready to pupate almost immediately after their deposition.

The proboscis is retracted into a pouch in the head at all times except when the insect is feeding (Fig. 68 A). Under these circumstances only its tip can be seen lying between the non-retractile maxillary palps. When protracted the proboscis extends well beyond the ends of the palps (Fig. 68 B). The mouthparts constituting the proboscis have a similar arrangement to those of *Glossina*, with the labellar lobes of the labium having eversible teeth and so being the organ of penetration. Both the labrum and the hypopharynx are located within the groove (gutter) of the labium (Fig. 68 C).

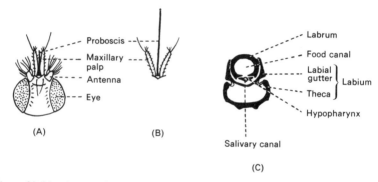

Figure 68 Mouthparts of *Pseudolynchia canariensis*: A, head and mouthparts, dorsal view showing proboscis retracted; B, proboscis protracted; C, transverse section through the proboscis.

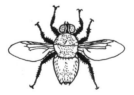

Figure 69 Adult *Hippobosca rufipes*.

Within the Hippoboscidae there are three important genera to be considered; they are *Hippobosca*, *Melophagus* and *Pseudolynchia*. The first of these genera contains *Hippobosca equina* and

H. rufipes, common parasites of equines and bovines in most warmer lands. The flies (Fig. 69) are approximately 10 to 12 mm long and are reddish-brown in colour with yellow spots. They have a single pair of wings and the venation is restricted to the anterior region, the remainder of the wing being completely devoid of veins (Fig. 70).

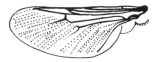

Figure 70 Wing of *Hippobosca rufipes*.

As indicated above, the female deposits larvae which she places singly into humus or dry soil. The larvae become puparia almost immediately and the adults emerge in the summer months. Once they have located a host they remain in position for long periods, usually occupying a site in either the inguinal region or on the hind legs. Although they are capable of extensive flight they seldom move more than a few yards and are transferred from one host to another by contact. Because they are nearly always located on the host they are relatively easily controlled by dipping.

Hippobosca species have been incriminated in the transmission of the blood parasites *Trypanosoma theileri* to cattle and *Haemoproteus* species to various ducks and other birds.

The genus *Melophagus* contains the keds, as, for example, *Melophagus ovinus*, the cosmopolitan 'sheep ked'. These are easily identified by their short, broad head, grey thorax, expanded brown abdomen and absence of wings (Fig. 71).

Each female produces between ten and fifteen larvae; these are cemented to the fleece of sheep. The larvae are ovoid and non-motile and pupate almost immediately to give rise to adults while still on the sheep. Adult keds suck blood from the sheep and cause irritation. In attempts to relieve themselves of the discomfort caused by the insects the sheep may scratch themselves and in so doing damage the fleece so causing economic loss. Also the faeces of keds discolour the wool and this is difficult to remove. It is the

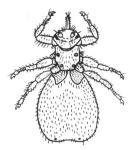

Figure 71 Adult *Melophagus ovinus.*

adult ked which is transferred from one host to another, and this is by direct contact of one sheep with another. Once again, because of their continuous presence on hosts keds may be successfully controlled by dipping.

Pseudolynchia species, for example *Pseudolynchia canariensis,* are similar to keds but possess wings (Fig. 72). Even so the wing venation is reduced and, as in *Hippobosca* species, the veins are found mostly on the fore parts of the wings. *Pseudolynchia canariensis* is distributed in the warmer countries of the world, being found on domesticated pigeons and a number of species of wild birds. It may also be found on humans who either keep pigeons as pets or come into close contact with wild birds.

Females produce only four or five larvae during their lives and deposit these on the birds when they are in their nests. As a result the larvae fall on to the nest material where they very soon become puparia.

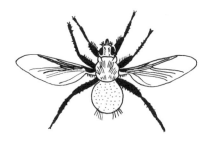

Figure 72 Adult *Pseudolynchia canariensis.*

Infected birds may be cured by application to the skin and feathers of a number of insecticide compounds such as derris.

Pseudolynchia canariensis has been shown to be a vector of both *Haemoproteus columbae* of pigeons and *H. lophortyx* of quail.

Horseflies

With the horse or gad flies (family Tabanidae) we pass from the suborder Cyclorrhapha to the suborder Brachycera. This taxonomic division contains just one family of parasitological importance, the members of which are large, heavily built flies which have powerful wings with a characteristic venation (Fig. 73) and are strong fliers. Their eyes are large and prominent and occupy most of the lateral regions of the head. The antennae are also robust and are

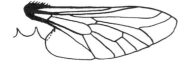

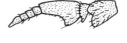

Figure 73 Wing of *Tabanus* species.   *Figure 74* Antenna of *Tabanus* species.

composed of two small proximal divisions and a third distally situated one which is large and subdivided (Fig. 74). In the genera *Tabanus* and *Chrysops* there are five subdivisions in the third antennal segment, in *Haematopota* there are four and in *Pangonia* seven to eight.

In some genera, for example *Tabanus* and *Haematopota*, the proboscis is quite short whilst in others, like *Chrysops* and *Pangonia*, it is elongated. Additionally, it is flexible and pendulant in *Tabanus, Chrysops* and *Haematopota* whilst in species of *Pangonia* it is forwardly directed. The labrum is relatively soft with a blunt tip and is not used in penetration. However, the mandibles are large and blade-like, and these and the styliform maxillary galeae are the piercing organs (Fig. 75). Once these mouthparts

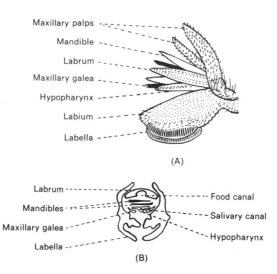

Maxillary palps
Mandible
Labrum
Maxillary galea
Hypopharynx
Labium
Labella

(A)

Labrum
Mandibles
Maxillary galea
Labella

Food canal
Salivary canal
Hypopharynx

(B)

Figure 75 Mouthparts of *Tabanus* species: A, lateral view of displayed mouthparts; B, transverse section through the proboscis at the level of the labellar lobes.

have made a wound and fluids are flowing out of it the labium, which does not enter the wound but kinks on the skin surface (see Fig. 132), draws up the blood by means of the pseudotracheae on the labellar lobes. Only the female tabanid imbibes blood, the male feeding exclusively on plant juices even though in possession of a full complement of mouthparts.

Female tabanids lay their eggs adjacent to water, quite often on vegetation which is overhanging water masses. Some 300 to 600 eggs are laid by each female and after four to seven days the caterpillar-like larvae (Fig. 76) hatch and drop into the water or mud along the edge. They enter the water and are most abundant in regions where there is a large amount of vegetation and the water is flowing slowly. The larva is composed of a head region which is difficult to distinguish and eleven body segments, each of which bears eight soft tubercles. Posteriorly there is a large, retractile air-tube through which the larva breathes. The larvae are carnivorous with powerful mandibles and feed on small invertebrates such as crustaceans. After several moults pupation

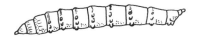

Figure 76 Larva of *Tabanus* species.

occurs in adjacent soil or mud and a few weeks are then required for the adult to emerge.

Adult flies are most numerous in the warmer months of the year and the females bite during daylight hours, especially on hot sultry days in dry wooded areas and along the sides of roads. They are severe and persistent biters causing annoyance and pain, and feed every two or three days on equines, deer, cattle and man. Several bites are usually necessary before they are fully engorged, after which they rest on nearby vegetation.

Control of tabanids is difficult, but measures have been devised to reduce the available breeding sites by drainage, to remove adult resting sites from the sides of roads and rivers, and to protect animals and people by the use of netting and by avoiding biting areas on hot, calm days.

As mentioned elsewhere, tabanids have been incriminated in the transmission of a number of diseases caused by bacteria and viruses, for example anthrax and tularaemia, the filarial disease loiasis, as well as several trypanosomes such as *Trypanosoma evansi evansi*, *T. equinum*, *T. vivax viennii*, *T. theileri* and all three *T. brucei* subspecies.

6

Fleas, lice and bugs

Fleas

The order Siphonaptera (= Aphaniptera) contains the common
mammal and bird parasites known as fleas. Unlike most other
ectoparasites they are laterally compressed, a feature which allows
them to pass freely between the hairs or feathers of their host.
Fleas have characteristically long legs which are directed beneath
the thorax and abdomen (Fig. 77). These are powerfully built and
are used to propel the insect forwards in a saltatory fashion, a
method of locomotion which is particularly effective in transferring

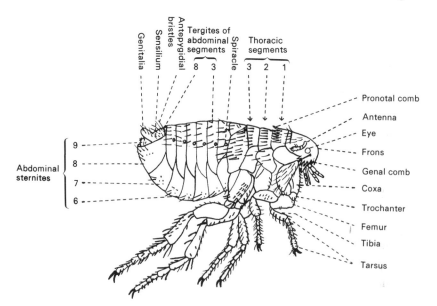

Figure 77 Common dog flea, *Ctenocephalides canis*, lateral view of male.

them from one host to another and in reaching a host from adjacent cover. The so-called human flea, *Pulex irritans*, has been shown to be capable of jumping in excess of 30 cm horizontally and nearly 20 cm vertically. Although not strictly a fair comparison, on a basis of size this would be equivalent to a human jumping 150 m and 90 m respectively. Arising from the body surface of a flea are numerous long setae, all of which are backwardly directed. These are consistent with forward progression through hairs and feathers and additionally prevent backward slip.

At this point, while discussing the locomotion and activity of fleas, it is necessary to draw attention to two important exceptions. They are the sticktight fleas, for example *Echidnophaga gallinacea* of poultry, and the chigoe or jigger flea, *Tunga penetrans*, a parasite of man and other mammals. Females of both of these species excavate their way into the skin of their host where they remain for most or all of their life.

On either side of the laterally compressed head of a flea there is a groove which houses a short, three-jointed antenna. In some species eyes are present, in which case they are located just in front of the antennae. Anteriorly the mouthparts are clearly visible. They comprise a pair of large, triangular maxillary stipites with associated long, four-jointed palps; a pair of styliform maxillary laciniae, often wrongly called the mandibles, which bear teeth along one edge; a slender labium with prominent two- to five-jointed palps; and a median, armed epipharynx (Fig. 78). Maxillary galeae and mandibles are absent, and the labrum is so small that it is difficult to distinguish.

By independent longitudinal movements the laciniae pierce the skin of the host and blood is drawn up by way of the channel formed by the apposition of the epipharynx and the laciniae under the influence of cibarial and pharyngeal suction pumps. Saliva is forced into the wound by a salivary pump, reaching the tissues through a canal formed between the laciniae (Fig. 78 D).

A peculiarity of the gut of fleas is the presence of circlets of backwardly directed spines arising from the inner wall of the proventriculus. Although their function has not been designated

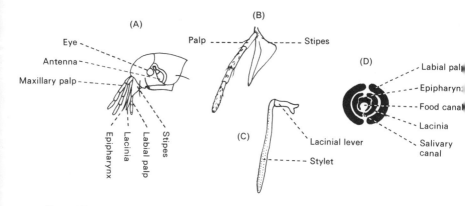

Figure 78 Head and mouthparts of a flea: A, head, lateral view; B, maxillary stipes and palp; C, maxillary lacinia; D, transverse section through the proboscis.

with certainty they probably act as valves and help in the mechanical breakdown of ingested corpuscles.

From the thoracic segments arise the legs which, as noted above, are long and powerful, with the hind legs being particularly elongated. At first sight it would appear that the flea has more podomeres to its limb than do other insects, but this is illusionary due to the fact that the coxae, which are poorly developed in most insects, are large and prominent and that the tarsi are five-jointed. Each limb ends in a pair of well-developed claws used in maintaining a hold on the substratum. Whereas the limbs are highly developed the wings are totally lacking. Thus fleas are good examples of insects in which the locomotory emphasis has been changed from the wings to the legs, in keeping with the requirements of its habits.

The abdomen is composed of ten segments, the last three of which are reduced and inconspicuous in females but which are modified in males to form claspers used during mating and an extremely complex penis, or aedaegus, which is retracted into the abdomen when not in use. The overall gross effect of such modification is that the tip of the male abdomen is upturned while it is rounded in the female. In cleared and mounted specimens of females the sclerotized seminal receptacle (spermatheca) is visible, the shape of which is of taxonomic value.

In both sexes the tergum of the tenth segment bears a sensory structure in the form of a pitted area together with a number of small setae. This is called the pygidium, or sensilium. Two other features useful in classification concerning setae are the long antepygidial bristles, between one and four pairs of which are found in most species, and the broad, closely arranged series of spines called combs, or ctenidia, located in some species on the gena of the head (genal comb), the dorsal surface of the first thoracic segment (pronotal comb) and occasionally on the abdomen. The presence or absence of these combs and their design is of particular value in diagnosis.

The life cycle of a flea involves both parasitic and free-living phases. Eggs are usually deposited indiscriminately a few at a time on to the bodies of the host but soon fall to the ground into nests or lairs or on floors of human dwellings. In all a female flea will lay between 300 and 500 eggs and in two to fourteen days these develop into legless larvae (Fig. 79 A) which feed on available organic debris and on the faeces of adult fleas which are rich in semi-digested blood. Flea larvae are somewhat caterpillar-like and most have dark heads and pale bodies. They are composed of fourteen segments, although one of these from the abdomen is not visible. A pair of small hooks called the anal struts are borne on the terminal segment and are employed in anchorage and as an aid to locomotion. About a week after hatching the larva is ready to pupate and prepares for this by forming a cocoon from pieces of

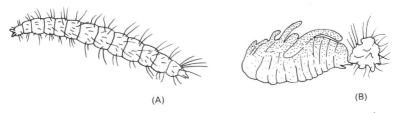

(A)   (B)

Figure 79 Immature stages of fleas, showing mature larva (A) and pupa removed from cocoon with larval exuvia still adhering to it (B).

debris, sand or other available material and sticking these together
with silken threads. Within the cocoon the larva pupates and
emerges some one to four weeks later as an adult flea. Having
emerged the adults seek a host on which to feed. Fleas are frequent
feeders and normally take a meal at least once per day, assuming
that hosts are readily available.

It is convenient to separate fleas into two superfamilies, namely
the Pulicoidea and the Ceratophylloidea. Many characteristics may
be used to distinguish between members of the two groupings,
among which are the absence of a vertical ridge on the outer
face of the mid-coxa and the presence of a maximum of one row
of setae on the terga of the abdominal segments in the Pulicoidea.
Such a ridge on the coxa is present in the Ceratophylloidea and
there is often more than one row of tergal setae. Of the genera
commonly affecting man and his domesticated animals *Tunga*,
Pulex, Xenopsylla, Ctenocephalides and *Echidnophaga* belong to
the Pulicoidea while *Nosopsyllus* is classified in the Ceratophylloidea.

Fleas are not host-specific although they do exhibit preferences
for certain animals. For this reason they may be particularly
troublesome to man for they are easily transferred to him from dogs,
cats and rats, in some cases disseminating diseases from the
reservoir to the human host. In the notes given below consideration
is given to some of the more important genera of fleas.

Pulex

Pulex irritans (Fig. 80 C) is the so-called human flea although it is
more commonly found on goats and pigs and is less frequently
encountered on foxes, badgers and man. It has virtually a
cosmopolitan geographical distribution although it is relatively rare
in tropical lands. The gut of *P. irritans* seldom becomes blocked
when infested with plague bacilli and thus this insect does not
rank among the important transmitters of plague.

Ctenocephalides

Essentially this genus belongs to the African continent although
certain species, for example *Ctenocephalides felis felis* (Fig. 80 E),

the cat flea, are cosmopolitan while *C. canis*, the dog flea, is now mainly Eurasian. Both of these insects may be associated with human habitations and are more important as human parasites than *Pulex irritans* as they are easily transferred from pets to man.

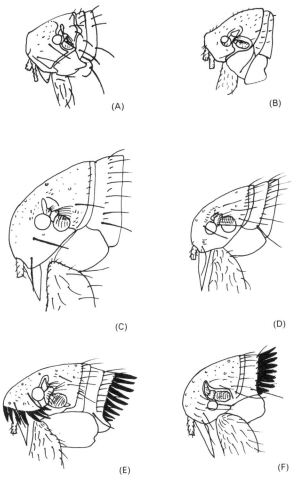

Figure 80 Heads of some common fleas : A, *Echidnophaga gallinacea* female, B, *Tunga penetrans* female ; C, *Pulex irritans* female ; D, *Xenopsylla cheopis* female ; E, *Ctenocephalides felis felis* female ; F, *Nosopsyllus fasciatus* female.

Xenopsylla

Although members of this genus are primarily Afroasian one important species, *Xenopsylla cheopis* (Fig. 80 D), has become distributed throughout the world accompanying its main host, the rat. It attacks man readily and is the chief vector of bubonic plague and murine typhus.

Echidnophaga

This is one of the genera of sticktight fleas, that is fleas in which the female penetrates into the skin and remains attached for most of her life. *Echidnophaga gallinacea* (Fig. 80 A), a common parasite of poultry with a worldwide distribution, is a serious pest and is easily transferred to mammals including man.

Tunga

The sand flea, jigger or chigoe, *Tunga penetrans* (Figs. 80 B and 81), of tropical Africa and America is so different from other fleas that a brief account of its life history is called for. The males are free-living and measure about 1 mm in length while the females are a little longer. After fertilization the female locates a host, which is

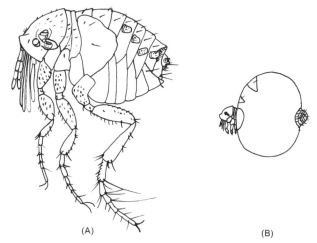

(A)   (B)

Figure 81 Female *Tunga penetrans*: A, unfed; B, fully fed. The two diagrams are drawn to a different scale.

often man, and burrows into the skin, usually under the nails of the feet. Here she resides, feeding and becoming enlarged to the size of a pea as the eggs develop within her body. The legs of the gravid female start to degenerate and the last two abdominal segments which do not increase in size protrude from the opening in the skin through which the insect gained entry. This permits the expulsion of the hundred or so eggs to the outside world. The eggs are about two-thirds the size of a virgin female and fall to the ground where they develop into larvae which feed on organic debris. Eventually they pupate within cocoons to give rise to the next generation adults.

When females are present in the skin a severe irritation may be experienced and the lesions may be painful and inflamed. Even when removed the wounds may become secondarily infected unless treated properly.

Nosopsyllus

Nosopsyllus fasciatus (Fig. 80 F) is another important vector of bubonic plague. It is the common rat flea in Europe and is found throughout the world, with a few notable exceptions such as India.

As mentioned elsewhere, as well as being pestiferous, fleas like *Xenopsylla cheopis* are responsible for the spread of a number of diseases including plague and murine typhus. In addition, fleas such as *Spilopsyllus cuniculi*, the European rabbit flea, transmit the causal agent of myxomatosis to rabbits while other species of fleas are responsible for disseminating the non-pathogenic rat trypanosome, *Trypanosoma lewisi*. Yet other fleas act as intermediate hosts of helminth parasites, among them the tapeworms *Dipylidium caninum* and *Hymenolepis diminuta*.

Fleas may be controlled by a number of chemical methods. While on their host, either rotenone or pyrethrum will kill them. These agents are safer to use than DDT and BHC which, although effective, may affect the host if licked off. The host's surroundings may also be treated to eliminate eggs and immature stages, and once again pyrethrum is effective.

Lice

There is no agreement as to whether the two types of lice, namely the sucking lice and the biting lice, should be considered as suborders—Siphunculata and Mallophaga respectively—of a single order, the Anoplura, or whether they should be allocated to separate orders—Anoplura and Mallophaga. In many respects the two types of lice are very similar, their main differences being concerned with the pattern of their mouthparts and methods of feeding. In the following account the latter means of classification is adopted.

Anoplura

The sucking lice are parasites of mammals only and are represented in the ectoparasitic fauna of man by the head louse, *Pediculus humanus humanus* (=*P. humanus capitis*), the body louse, *P. humanus corporis* (Fig. 82), and the crab, or pubic, louse, *Phthirus pubis* (Fig. 83). Occasionally the pig louse, *Haematopinus suis*, has been recorded from man, but this is best considered as an accidental parasite. Other important parasites of animals frequently encountered are *Linognathus pedalis*, the foot louse of sheep, and *Haematopinus asini*, of horses.

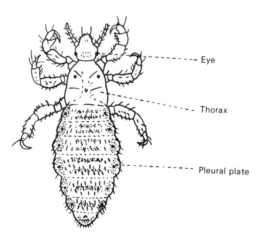

Figure 82 Pediculus humanus adult, the human louse.

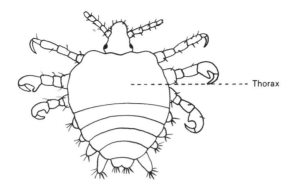

Figure 83 Adult *Phthirus pubis*, the pubic or crab louse.

As indicated above, the main differences between sucking and biting lice are to be found in the mouthparts. In contrast to the Mallophaga, sucking lice do not possess functional mandibles, but have piercing stylets and are equipped with well-developed suctorial pumps.

The mouthparts (Fig. 84) are extremely modified and the homologies of the parts are still debated by many authors. The proboscis is short and comprises a labrum armed with recurved teeth, which is used for anchorage into the wound, and three stylets. The dorsal stylet, thought by the majority to be a derivative of the hypopharynx and by some to be the maxilla, encloses the food canal. Below this is the intermediate or median stylet, a slender tube, the lumen of which is the salivary canal. It is presumed that this is also a development from the hypopharynx. The most ventrally situated stylet, likely derived from the labium, is the main organ of penetration and has a toothed apex. Both the maxillae and the mandibles are very much reduced. They merge with the lateral walls of the pre-oral food canal and are not obvious as individual mouthparts.

Once the ventral stylet has pierced the skin and the remaining mouthparts have gained entry, the fluids are sucked into the gut by both cibarial and pharyngeal pumps. There is no salivary pump to aid in the ejection of the salivary secretion.

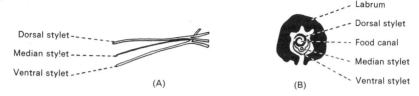

Figure 84 Mouthparts of Anoplura : A, stylets dissected out ; B, transverse section through the proboscis.

In most sucking lice the eyes are either small or absent. However, in the human parasites they are not only present but are quite well developed. Just in front of the eyes are located the antennae, which are normally composed of five divisions.

The thorax is small and all three segments are fused together. It bears six relatively short legs, each ending in a single claw which may be opposed to a projection on the tibia giving an efficient organ for holding on to hairs of the host (Fig. 85). In common with the fleas, wings are completely absent in these insects. The relatively large abdomen is composed of nine segments, only seven of which are apparent. On the lateral regions of these segments dark chitinous plates are present; these are known as paratergal, or pleural, plates, the significance of which is obscure.

Phthirus pubis may be encountered on hairs of the pubic and perianal regions, and occasionally on hairs of the face, armpits and other regions, either together with or in the absence of pubic infestation. It has a broad, short, grey body and long, red legs, the first pair of which is noticeably smaller than the remaining two.

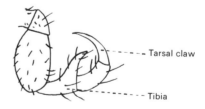

Figure 85 Front leg of a male *Pediculus humanus corporis*, showing the tarsal claw which opposes a process of the tibia.

Female pubic lice usually measure between 1·5 and 2·0 mm in
length while the males are somewhat smaller.

Eggs are laid in batches of from twenty to thirty, each being
glued to a body hair. About a week later they hatch to first-stage
nymphs which moult to second- and third-stage nymphs prior to
becoming adults some two or three weeks after hatching. Adults
live for a few weeks only and are passed from one person to
another by contact, usually venereally—hence the common name
for this cosmopolitan louse of 'papillon d'amour'.

The human body and head lice, *Pediculus humanus corporis* and
P. humanus humanus, also enjoy a cosmopolitan geographical
distribution. As far as their occurrence on man is concerned, the
body louse is found on the body only whereas the latter subspecies
is distributed on both the head and the body. The two subspecies
are morphologically very similar although specimens of *humanus*
are slightly smaller (females measure 2·4 to 3·3 mm in length),
have shorter antennal podomeres (Fig. 86) and are brown in colour,
compared with specimens of *corporis*, the females of which are 2·4
to 3·8 mm long, have longer antennal divisions and are grey. In
both cases the females are slightly larger than the males.

Eggs of *P. humanus humanus* (Fig. 87) are cemented to hairs by

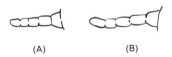

(A) (B)

Figure 86 Antennae of A, *Pediculus humanus humanus* and B, *P. humanus corporis.*

a sticky secretion whereas those of *P. humanus corporis* are glued
to the fibres of clothing. In both subspecies the eggs are very large
(approximately 1 mm long) and it has been estimated that female
body lice lay about 300 eggs whereas female head lice produce
only 100. The eggs, which are commonly known as 'nits', hatch
into first-instar nymphs in about ten days in warm conditions, and
these feed in a similar fashion to the adults. As usual, three
nymphal instars occur in the life cycle and the final-stage nymph
moults to give an adult. Between two and four weeks elapse from

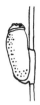

Figure 87 Egg (nit) of *Pediculus humanus humanus* attached to a hair.

hatching to the formation of the imago. Adults live for a short time only, with four to six weeks being quoted for females, males living a slightly shorter time.

Head and body lice must feed every two or three days under conditions of high temperature, although at low temperatures they can survive for up to ten days without a blood meal. Lice do not become replete when they feed, but given an adequate supply of hosts will imbibe small volumes of blood several times a day. Whereas head lice are found on the body and feed while holding on to the skin surface, body lice usually hold on to clothing with their hind legs and reach across to the adjacent skin to feed. Thus body lice are quite likely to be encountered on clothing rather than on the body surface itself.

Unless dislodged, lice remain on the host and are transferred from one host to another either by direct contact, where one person touches another, or by indirect contact, for example when someone uses a comb or clothing of an infested person.

Pediculus humanus subspecies may spread skin disorders mechanically by carrying the disease-causing organisms on their bodies and legs. An example of a disease so spread is impetigo. In addition, these lice have been shown to transmit the aetiological agents of relapsing fever, typhus fever and trench fever cyclically, as discussed in chapter 11. Other effects of lice on their hosts are dealt with at the end of this chapter.

Mallophaga

Members of this group of lice are parasitic on birds mainly. There are a few species found on mammals but none is indigenous to the primates. Mallophaga are commonly called bird lice or chewing lice, and as the latter name would indicate they feed on feathers, hairs, epithelial debris and in some cases tissue fluids and blood which they make available by masticatory actions.

Biting lice are small, dorso-ventrally flattened insects which lack wings and have short legs with two tarsal claws in the bird parasites and only one in species parasitic on mammals. The second and third segments of the thorax are always fused together, but the prothoracic segment is free, thus giving the appearance of a thorax of two divisions only. The abdomen may be either broad or narrow, depending upon the species, and nine segments are normally apparent.

Biting lice are divided into two suborders, the main characteristics which separate them being connected with the appendages of the head.

1 *Amblycera*   These are bird and mammal parasites with short antennae, usually of four divisions, housed in grooves on the undersurface of the head. They possess maxillary palps and the mandibles move in a plane parallel with the underside of the head, that is they bite horizontally.

2 *Ischnocera*   Again these are found on both birds and mammals, but have antennae of three to five divisions projecting freely from the lateral surfaces of the head. They do not have maxillary palps and the mandibles are suspended from the head such that the bite is vertical.

The heads of all biting lice are large and often broad. From the head arise the characteristic mouthparts, the most conspicuous of which are the large biting mandibles equipped with teeth and the broad plate-like labium which separates the maxillae (Fig. 88). Only on close examination can the hypopharynx be seen, and this is drawn out into two long forwardly projecting filaments, the function of which is still uncertain although they may aid the mandibles in abrading tissues. In the main, biting lice feed by cutting off lengths of either hairs or feathers with the mandibles, although reports of feeding on skin secretions and debris are common.

The life cycles of biting lice are similar to those of sucking lice with the insects remaining on the host unless transferred by contact to another animal. The eggs are glued to either feathers or hairs and

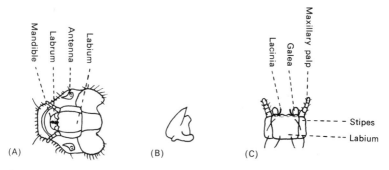

Figure 88 Head and mouthparts of Mallophaga (Amblycera) : A, ventral view of head ; B, right mandible, ventral view ; C, labium and maxillae, ventral view.

hatch in from three to five days to give a first-stage nymph. Three moults and two to four weeks later the imaginal instar is reached.

Among the important species of Mallophaga are *Cuclotogaster heterographus*, the head louse of poultry; *Trichodectes canis* of dogs, which is an intermediate host of the tapeworm *Dipylidium canium*; *Felicola subrostratus* of cats; *Damalinia bovis* of cattle (Fig. 89 A) and *D. equi* of horses; and *Columbicola columbae* of pigeons (Fig. 89 D), all of which are grouped in the Ischnocera. There are, in addition, a number of important members of the Amblycera, notably *Menopon gallinae*, the shaft louse of poultry, ducks and pigeons (Fig. 89 C) and *Heterodoxus spiniger* of dogs.

Effects of lice on their hosts
As they crawl over the surface of an animal, lice may cause intense irritation. This makes the host animal restless such that it scratches fiercely and bites itself so abrading and damaging its coat. Sometimes animals may swallow large amounts of hair as they bite

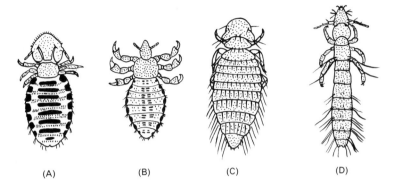

Figure 89 Representative cattle and bird lice : A, *Damalinia bovis* from cattle (Mallophaga) ; B, *Haematopinus eurysternus* from cattle (Anoplura) ; C, *Menopon gallinae* from chickens (Mallophaga) ; D, *Columbicola columbae* from pigeons (Mallophaga).

at their coats which may disrupt their normal digestive activities. Skin lesions lead to substantial economic losses by the destruction of hides and damage to wool, and the wounds may become infected with bacteria so causing even more discomfort to the animals. In addition to this, the excretory products of lice may discolour wool such that expensive cleaning processes are necessary before the product is usuable.

Apart from these primary effects of louse bites there are, of course, a number of diseases transmitted both mechanically and cyclically, as mentioned elsewhere.

Control of lice
All lice may be controlled by similar treatment. In the case of poultry and domesticated birds the application of strong tobacco extract containing about 40 per cent nicotine to bird houses and cages is recommended, as is the dusting of such places with BHC and the use of dust baths containing $\frac{1}{2}$ per cent lindane. This latter treatment is especially useful as it kills many other ectoparasites, including ticks and mites.

Cattle, sheep and dogs may be treated with dips containing low concentrations of BHC, but such treatment is not to be recommended for cats as chlorinated hydrocarbons are particularly toxic to them. Instead, dusting with 3 per cent rotenone powder is effective.

Humans may also be treated with chlorinated hydrocarbons, the first choice usually being DDT powder at a concentration of about 10 per cent. Should this fail to kill the lice due to their resistance to the compound, then 1 per cent lindane powder may be used.

Bugs

The order Hemiptera contains the true bugs, all of which possess piercing and sucking mouthparts. Whilst the majority of members of the group abstract fluids from plants and other insects, a few have become parasitic on higher animals.

Taxonomically the bugs are of two types: Homoptera, with both pairs of wings membranous, and Heteroptera, with the basal parts of the forewings of a tougher texture than the terminal regions and with the hindwings uniformly membranous. Such forewings are known as hemelytra.

Only two families of bugs, the Cimicidae (bed-bugs) and the Reduviidae (assassin bugs) concern the parasitologist, both of which are heteropterans. Many other bugs such as aphids, mealy bugs and scale insects are also of great economic importance as they feed on plants and crops and so affect man in yet another way.

Bed-bugs

The common bed-bug is *Cimex lectularius* (Fig. 90), an insect some 4 to 5 mm long which attacks man, domesticated animals and poultry in temperate regions of the world. In the tropics it is replaced by an allied species, *C. hemipterus*, which it resembles closely but from which it can be distinguished by the shape of the head and anterior region of the thorax (Fig. 91). Bed-bugs have broad, dorso-ventrally flattened bodies which are covered with bristles. They are elongated oval in shape and reddish-brown in colour.

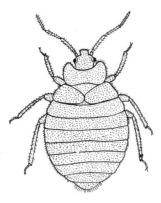

Figure 90 Adult male *Cimex lectularius*, the bed-bug.

From the head arise a pair of long four-jointed antennae, the basal joints of which are much smaller than the others. Also prominent are the two compound eyes which project from the lateral parts of the head. The head is set deeply into the prothorax and the pronotum is expanded laterally to, in part, surround the sides of the head. The second thoracic segment, the mesothorax, bears the wing pads, the non-functional vestiges of the flying apparatus which almost completely hide the notum of the metathorax. Six legs are associated with the thorax and each is equipped with a terminal claw. Although the legs have the normal complement of podomeres they have more than the basic number of divisions as the tarsi are three-jointed. The first and second

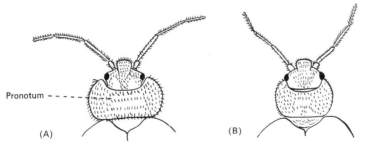

Figure 91 Dorsal views of the anterior regions of *Cimex lectularius*, the common bed-bug of temperate regions (A) and *C. hemipterus*, the tropical bed-bug (B).

segments of the abdomen are fused together while the third to the ninth are visible as distinct entities. This gives the overall impression of an abdomen with eight divisions. In the male the tip of the abdomen is pointed whilst in the female it is rounded, a characteristic which serves to give a useful means of separating the sexes on superficial examination.

From the head arise the mouthparts (Fig. 92) comprising a broad, triangular labrum, a prominent four-jointed labium which is hollowed to accommodate a pair of mandibular and a pair of maxillary stylets, equivalent to the galeae. Both a food canal and a salivary canal are formed between the interlocked maxillary stylets (Fig. 92 E). A small, flattened, triangular hypopharynx is also present but does not contribute to the proboscis.

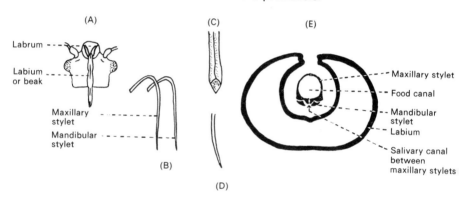

Figure 92 Head and mouthparts of Heteroptera: A, head, ventral view; B, mandibular and maxillary stylets dissected out; C, tip of maxillary stylets showing interlocked position; D, tip of a mandibular stylet; E, transverse section through the proboscis.

The stylets are capable of protraction and retraction, and by their repeated movement puncture the surface of the host. Both of the mandibular stylets are equipped with denticles at their apices and aid in penetration as well as preventing the bug from being dislodged from the skin when attached. When the bug is feeding the stylets are driven into the skin whilst the labium bends backwards. Fluids from the host are subsequently drawn up into the gut by means of a cibarial pump, there being no pharyngeal

pump. Salivary secretion is meanwhile being forcibly ejected into
the wound by a pump housed in the hypopharynx. The secretion
reaches the skin via a canal which opens at the tip of the
hypopharynx and a channel in the maxillary stylets.

Bites of bed-bugs may cause considerable irritation and
discomfort and may, under certain circumstances, lead to anaemia,
palpitation of the heart and eye troubles when an excessive
number of bites are experienced. As far as is known, bed-bugs are
not responsible for the dissemination of disease under natural
conditions. However like almost any other haematophagous insect
they can transmit mechanically if disturbed while feeding on an
infected host and allowed to continue feeding on another host.
Although bed-bugs defaecate after feeding and so are potentially
capable of transmitting disease by contamination, they often remain
on clothing when they bite and reach across to the skin to feed. It
thus follows that the excrement is usually deposited on the clothing
rather than near to the wound. This may well explain why bed-bugs
are not involved in disease transmission.

Feeding takes place at night, the bugs leaving their hideouts to
bite their sleeping hosts. On average they take from ten to fifteen
minutes to become replete before retreating to their hiding places
which are cracks and crevices in furniture, beddings and walls in
human dwellings. It must be appreciated that unfed bugs are
flattened and so can enter very thin cracks but that when replete
their choice of retreat is more restricted.

Having imbibed sufficient blood for egg maturation to commence
a female returns to her crevice to lay one or two eggs per day until
she has produced a total of 100 to 200 operculate eggs (Fig. 93 A).

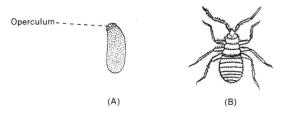

Operculum- - - - - - -

(A)   (B)

Figure 93 Cimex lectularius: A, egg; B, newly hatched nymph.

These hatch after four to twelve days in warm weather to a first-nymphal instar (Fig. 93 B) which, in common with the succeeding four nymphal stages, feeds on blood. Under warm conditions about eight to ten weeks pass from hatching until the fifth-nymphal stage develops into an adult.

Animals serve as a food source only for bed-bugs, and it is important to realize that hosts do not carry bugs from place to place but that they are spread by furniture and bedding which is moved from one human dwelling to another. Dieldrin, lindane, DDT and BHC have all been usefully employed against these pests and are best applied to furniture, bedding and cracks and crevices in walls in places where the bugs are known to exist.

Assassin bugs

These large, brightly coloured insects belong to the family Reduviidae, subfamily Triatominae, and so are referred to as either triatomid or reduviid bugs. Other names designated to them are cone-nosed bugs because of the shape of their anterior extremity and kissing bugs on account of their habit of biting people on and around the face.

An assassin bug (Fig. 94) is easily identified by its narrow head from which emerges a pair of very long four-jointed antennae and a strong three-jointed labium (Fig. 95) housing the remainder of the mouthparts. The proboscis curves backwards when the insect is not feeding to lie against the body with its tip in a hollow of the

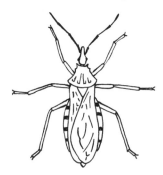

Figure 94 Adult *Triatoma megista*, an assassin bug.

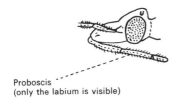

Proboscis
(only the labium is visible)

Figure 95 Lateral view of the head of *Triatoma megista.*

prosternum. The mouthparts are of similar design to those of bed-bugs and inflict bites which are not only painful but which are sometimes dangerous causing severe allergic reactions.

Behind the head the pronotum is expanded posteriorly and is subdivided into an anterior and a posterior region by a suture line. Just posterior to the pronotum the scutellum can be seen and is quite often drawn out into a posterior spine. The lateral margins of the abdomen are distinctly compressed and are not overlaid by the wings when the insect is at rest. These regions of the abdomen as well as the thickened parts of the hemelytra and the dorsal surface of the thorax are usually brightly coloured. In *Rhodnius prolixus* they are brown and yellow and in *Panstrongylus megistus* red and black.

Reduviid bugs are especially abundant in warmer parts of the world, although a few species are almost cosmopolitan in their geographical distribution. Of these only a few species feed on blood, including that of man, and attack at night when the host is resting. Assassin bugs are usually not very host-specific, although a few species such as *Rhodnius prolixus, Panstrongylus megistus* and *Triatoma infestans* are always associated with human habitations and so feed mainly on human blood. Such species are found in cracks and crevices of walls by day and emerge only at night to feed.

In common with other bugs metamorphosis is gradual. The eggs are usually oviposited singly or in small batches, although *Rhodnius prolixus* is exceptional in that it produces large masses. A total of 100 to 300 eggs are laid and these require two to three weeks to hatch into wingless first-instar nymphs. The immature stages are all blood-feeders and after gaining sufficient nutriment the nymphs moult. In all there are five nymphal stages and the wings gradually develop as the insect passes through successive moults. The time taken for the life cycle to be completed from egg to adult varies with environmental conditions, but approximates to a year and a half.

Triatomid bugs are disease-transmitters, with many *Rhodnius* species being responsible for the spread of *Trypanosoma rangeli* and species such as *Rhodnius prolixus, Panstrongylus megistus* and *Triatoma infestans* disseminating *Trypanosoma cruzi*. Of the carriers of the latter flagellate, *R. prolixus* is common in northern South America and in Central America, *P. megistus* in most of Brazil and *T. infestans* in parts of Brazil as well as in Argentina, Bolivia, Chile, Paraguay and Uraguay. *T. cruzi* is transmitted exclusively by the contamination of wounds by the faeces of the bug, and so it is a prerequisite for the transmission of this parasite that the insect defaecates either during or immediately after feeding while still on the host.

Reduviids are much more difficult to control than bed-bugs because of their activity. They are not only strong fliers with well-developed wings but are also good runners and nearly always avoid capture. It is possible to prevent their entry into dwellings using nets, and species associated with houses may be eradicated with either BHC or dieldrin sprays or by plastering walls so that hiding places are not available to the bugs.

7
Bot flies and warble flies

Larvae of members of the dipteran families Gasterophilidae and Oestridae, the bot flies and warble flies respectively, are normally parasitic in domesticated animals. This parasitism is an example of myiasis (see also chapter 5) and causes severe discomfort to animals and considerable economic loss to man.

The Gasterophilidae contains only one genus, *Gasterophilus*, which is divided into a number of species, all of which are parasitic in equines and, occasionally, dogs, pigs and man. Adult flies are large (18 mm long) and hairy and superficially resemble bees, although of course they possess only a single pair of wings. The mouthparts of the flies are vestigial and hence they are unable to feed, all of their required nutrients being derived from foodstores built up during the immature stages.

G. intestinalis is the most common species of the genus, an adult of which is depicted in Fig. 96 showing the characteristic broad, dark bands which traverse each wing. The adults are short-lived and the female lays her eggs during the latter months of summer, cementing them to hairs on the body of the host (Fig. 97). The

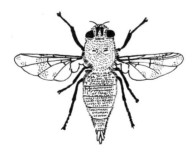

Figure 96 Adult *Gasterophilus intestinalis*.

Figure 97 Egg of *Gasterophilus intestinalis.*

precise site of oviposition depends on the species of bot fly. Thus in *G. intestinalis* it is the forelegs, in *G. nasalis* the chin and throat and in *G. inermis* and *G. haemorrhoidalis* the region surrounding the mouth. Of the *Gasterophilus* species, *G. pecorum* is exceptional in that, although eggs may be laid on the hoofs and lower legs of the host, they are usually deposited on fodder and in pastures (Fig. 98). When eggs are laid in the vicinity of the mouth they hatch spontaneously as soon as the larvae have developed within the egg membranes. In other cases the eggs require to be licked before hatching will occur. In either set of circumstances the larvae enter the mouth of the host and burrow into the tissues of the oral

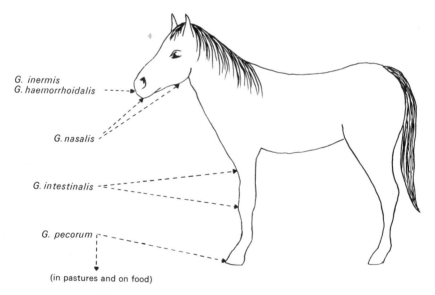

Figure 98 Site of egg deposition of *Gasterophilus* species.

mucosa. Here they remain for some two to four weeks but give rise
to little or no host reaction. Eventually they leave this site and pass
down the alimentary canal to attach to another region of the gut
surface. Once again the site parasitized varies with the species. It is
the stomach in *G. intestinalis* and *G. haemorrhoidalis*, either the
stomach or the duodenum in *G. nasalis*, and the pharynx and
oesophagus (site of second-stage larva) and the stomach (third-
stage larva) in *G. pecorum*. No matter which gut region is selected
lesions are produced by the larvae and the resultant exudates are
used as a food source. The host responds to this tissue damage
with inflammatory reactions.

Larvae remain within their host for about a year and, in the
following spring, they leave the alimentary canal as third-stage
larvae together with faecal materials. In *G. haemorrhoidalis* the
larvae do not pass straight out but reattach to the rectal wall for a
few days before their eventual departure. The third-stage larva is
quite characteristic and easy to recognize (Fig. 99 A). It has twelve
segments, the first two of which are fused together, and has one
(*G. nasalis*) or two circlets of spines on most of these. *G. inermis*
differs from other bot flies in that spines are lacking from its cuticle.
The posterior spiracular plates help in identification for they are
unique in being fused together and having six curved spiracular
slits (Fig. 99 B). In the first-stage larva the fused plate has only
two slits and in the second-stage larva it has four.

Having left the equine host the larvae pupate in the ground and
some four or five weeks later become adults. The adult flies cause
the equine to become disturbed and make it irritable and restless.
In most cases the larvae cause little harm although inflammatory
responses in the form of severe ulceration may be seen in gut

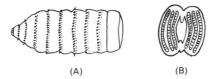

(A)   (B)

Figure 99 Third-stage larva of *Gasterophilus intestinalis* (A). Fused spiracular plates
of larva (B).

tissues as a result of local lesions caused by the abrasive spines and the mouth-hooks. When present in large numbers the larvae may interfere with the normal passage of food products through the alimentary canal, and in some hosts it is believed that a hyper-sensitive reaction may be initiated by the excretory products of larvae which are voided into the gut lumen and subsequently absorbed into the host's body.

Larvae which are in the stomach may be killed by the administration of either carbon tetrachloride or carbon bisulphide, while the host may be freed of eggs by either regular grooming or the application of carbolic to the coat.

Adult members of the Oestridae (the warble and nasal flies), like the Gasterophilidae, are large, hairy, bee-like flies with rudimentary mouthparts. Unlike the bot flies, however, the larvae of Oestridae are parasitic either beneath the skin or within the body cavities of mammals. The family contains four genera of importance: *Oestrus*, *Hypoderma*, *Dermatobia* and *Cuterebra*.

The sheep nasal fly, *Oestrus ovis*, occurs not only in sheep but also in goats and man. The adult (Fig. 100) is about 12 mm long

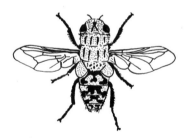

Figure 100 Adult *Oestrus ovis.*

and has prominent black spots on its body surface. It is short-lived and is found in the summer when the female, which is larviparous, deposits larvae into and around the nostrils of a host. The larvae eventually enter the nasal passages and moult to second- and later third-stage larvae. They leave the host from three to twelve months after their arrival, the emergent third-stage larva being pale in colour but with dark bands traversing the dorsal region of the majority of

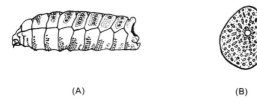

(A) (B)

Figure 101 Third-stage larva of *Oestrus ovis* (A) and spiracular plate of larva (B).

its segments. It is about 30 mm long with well-developed mouth-hooks, rows of small spines on the ventral surface and characteristic spiracular plates (Fig. 101). Out of the host the larvae drop to the ground to pupate and after four to six weeks the adults emerge.

The flies cause great annoyance to sheep, which take evasive action by pushing their noses either into each other's fleece or into the ground. This interferes with their feeding and has effects on the economics of farming. Inside the nasal cavities the larvae cause irritation which produces copious mucous secretions accompanied by sneezing. It is on these secretions that the larvae feed.

Although it is difficult to prevent sheep nasal flies from depositing their larvae on sheep, the anointing of tar around the nasal region of the animals is useful. The administration of various organophosphorous compounds has been shown to clear up existing infections of larvae quite efficiently.

Throughout the northern hemisphere the ox warble flies, *Hypoderma bovis* and *H. lineatum*, can be found. They commonly infect cattle, but additionally occur in horses and man although complete development does not take place in the equine and human species.

The flies are approximately 12 mm long and are banded with yellow and black stripes (Fig. 102). The short-lived adults emerge in summer and lay their several hundred eggs fixed to hairs, usually those on the legs, by means of terminal clasps. In the case of *H. bovis* the eggs are laid singly whilst in *H. lineatum* they are deposited in rows of a half a dozen or more (Fig. 103). Less than a week after being laid the eggs hatch and the larvae burrow through the skin and wander in the subcutaneous connective tissues up the

H

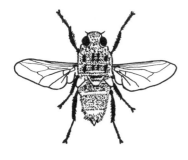

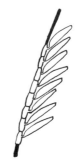

Figure 103 Eggs of Hypoderma lineatum
Figure 102 Adult Hypoderma bovis.   attached to a hair.

leg towards the animal's back. In the case of H. lineatum the larvae
enter the wall of the oesophagus where they remain until early in
the next year before continuing their journey towards the dorsum.
In contrast, H. bovis larvae usually follow the path of a nerve from
the skin and so enter the spinal cord. They remain in this organ for
a short time only before proceeding to the muscles of the back.
During their migrations Hypoderma larvae moult once and then
moult again when they arrive at the dorsum to give a third-stage
larva which is about 25 to 40 mm long with several small spines
and tubercles on most of its segments (Fig. 104 A). The
protuberances are absent from the last segment in H. lineatum and
from the last two segments in H. bovis. In addition to the above
features positive identification of the larva may be made by means
of the shape of the posterior spiracles (Fig. 104 B).

A swelling approximately 25 mm in diameter marks the position
of each larva. Within each cyst the larva lies with its spiracles
pushed through a perforation in the skin to respire. Larvae remain in

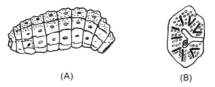

(A)   (B)

Figure 104 Third-stage larva of Hypoderma bovis (A) and spiracular plates of
larva (B).

these locations for a month or so, feeding on blood and tissue exudates, and at the end of this period of time, which coincides with the spring, the third-stage larva leaves the host to pupate on the ground and become an adult. About four or five weeks are required for pupation.

The flies are extremely persistent in their attempts to lay eggs and cause the cattle great distress, making the animals run to avoid them. Quite often the animals collide with objects and hurt themselves and many become exhausted. As the larvae excavate tissue reactions occur, but are unimportant compared with the swellings on the backs which are troublesome to the cattle and cause great economic loss due to the destruction of hides.

Treatment involves the administration of organophosphorous compounds which kill migrating larvae as well as those in surface cysts. Troublesome fully formed larvae may also be removed surgically.

Dermatobia hominis is another large fly and can be identified by its characteristic blue body and brown wings. It is found in Central and South America and the larvae parasitize a variety of animals including cattle, equines, dogs and man. When the female fly is about to lay her eggs she catches a blood-sucking insect, usually a mosquito of the genus *Psorophora*, although other mosquitoes and *Stomoxys* species will serve the purpose. The female *Dermatobia* then cements about a dozen eggs to the venter of the transport insect and when it feeds on its host the eggs, if fully developed, hatch when stimulated by the skin temperature. The larvae crawl on to the integument of the mammal and penetrate it, quite often through the lesion produced by the feeding mosquito. Within the skin the larvae grow and moult, and a cyst slowly develops around them, the swelling protruding from the surface of the body. Within the cyst the larva lies with its posterior spiracles pushed through an aperture. Eventually the third-stage larva, which has characteristic rows of spines on most of its segments and which measures about 25 mm in length (Fig. 105), leaves the host to pupate on the ground, and in one to two and a half months the adult fly emerges.

The cysts are painful and it is often necessary to remove larvae

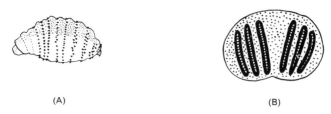

Figure 105 Third-stage larva of *Dermatobia hominis* (A) and fused spiracular plates of larva (B).

from the skin surgically. The dipping of cattle in washes containing insecticides like BHC and DDT is another useful treatment.

In North America *Cuterebra* species are found, the larvae of which are parasitic in the subcutaneous tissues of small mammals and occasionally dogs, cats and man. The females lay their eggs at the openings of lagomorph and rodent burrows and the emergent larvae penetrate into the skin of rabbits, in the case of *C. lepivora*, or chipmunks and mice, in *C. emasculator*. About a month after penetration a cyst develops around each fully formed larva. This maggot is between 15 and 30 mm long and has large black spines on most of its segments. Eventually each larva leaves the host to pupate on the ground and become an imago.

Little success has been obtained in the chemotherapeutic treatment of cysts caused by *Cuterebra* species and the only really proven treatment is to remove them individually using surgical methods.

Part II
Biology of the pathogens

8

Malaria and other mosquito-borne diseases

Of all the insects known to man the mosquito is unquestionably the one which causes most illness, economic loss and discomfort. Many mosquitoes transmit diseases which affect man and his domesticated stock, among the more important of which are malaria, filariasis, yellow fever, dengue and various forms of virus disease. Even when they do not disseminate disease, mosquitoes may cause great annoyance and make areas otherwise suitable for human and animal occupation quite uninhabitable.

Malaria

The name 'malaria' has been used to describe a variety of diseases but is here employed in a restricted and widely accepted fashion for the disease caused by species of the genus *Plasmodium*. Members of this protozoan genus occur in reptiles, birds and mammals only, with man being a susceptible host to a number of species. The malarial parasites have been classified in various ways, and even today alternative schemes exist. Some authorities regard all malarial parasites to be members of the family Haemoproteidae, while others consider there to be three separate groupings:

$$
\text{Family Haemoproteidae} = \begin{cases} \text{Family Plasmodiidae containing the single} \\ \quad \text{genus } \textit{Plasmodium} \\ \text{Family Haemoproteidae, e.g. } \textit{Haemoproteus} \\ \text{Family Leucocytozoidae, e.g. } \textit{Leucocytozoon} \end{cases}
$$

Species of the genus *Plasmodium* are obligate parasites and are intracellular for most of their life cycle, which is spent partly in a vertebrate and partly in a mosquito. Within the mosquito sexual

109

reproduction takes place while in the vertebrate host multiplication is asexual and occurs by a process known as schizogony. This method of reproduction involves the growth of a cell followed by the division of its nucleus before the cytoplasm has been aportioned. Finally the cytoplasm is split to form numerous uninucleate individuals called merozoites. Cycles of schizogony occur inside the red blood corpuscles (erythrocytes) of the host and within other body tissues.

Other characteristics of malarial parasites which deserve mention are that the gametocytes, or gamete precursors, occur in the circulating red blood corpuscles of the host, from which site they are taken up by feeding female mosquitoes, and that the individuals located within erythrocytes are pigmented. This is due to the fact that the parasites metabolize haemoglobin from the host corpuscle, digesting the protein to obtain amino acids and storing the waste fraction in vacuoles in the cytoplasm. The waste product is dark in colour and is referred to as haemozoin, or malarial pigment. Haemoglobin provides the malarial parasite with all of the necessary amino acids except for methionine which, together with glucose, is obtained from the corpuscle via the plasma. The glucose is used to provide energy by its oxidation to carbon dioxide and water (Kreb's cycle), while the amino acids are utilized primarily for growth.

Subdivisions of the genus
It is convenient to subdivide the genus *Plasmodium* into a number of subgenera, as shown in Table 3.

Life cycles (Fig. 106)
The life cycles of all members of the genus, irrespective of their subgenus, are extremely similar, as is shown in the following account.

The stage infective to the vertebrate is a small, elongated uninucleate body called a sporozoite, many of which are introduced into the blood of a host together with salivary secretions when an infected female mosquito feeds. The sporozoites circulate in the

Table 3 Subdivisions of the genus *Plasmodium*

Subgenus	Vectors	Vertebrate host	Erythro-cytic schizonts	Gameto-cytes	Other characteristics
Plasmodium	⎫	⎫ primates	large	round	⎛ e.e.c. * in liver par-
Laverania	⎬	⎬	large	cres-centic	⎪ enchyma only ; no
	⎬ Anopheles	⎭			⎨ secondary e.e.c. in
	⎬	lemurs and			⎝ *Laverania*
Vinckeia	⎭	non-primate mammals	small	round	⎰ e.e.c. in liver ⎱ parenchyma only
Haemamoeba	⎫ various	⎫	large	round	⎛ primary e.e.c. in
Huffia	⎬ anopheline	⎬ birds	large	elongate	⎪ lymphoid-
Giovannolaia	⎨ and culicine	⎬	large	elongate	⎨ macrophage cells
Novyella	⎬ mosquitoes	⎭	small	elongate/oval	⎪ of skin; secondary
	⎬				⎪ e.e.c. in lymphoid
Sauramoeba	⎬ unknown	⎫ reptiles	large	elongate	⎪ macrophage cells
Carinia	⎭	⎭	small	elongate/oval	⎝ anywhere in body

*e.e.c. = exoerythrocytic cycle

blood-stream for about half an hour and then penetrate tissue cells where they grow and then multiply by schizogony. The sporozoites are, in fact, well adapted for penetration and possess complex anterior organelles thought to produce histolytic secretions and numerous mitochondria and peripheral contractile fibres to permit locomotion.

Variation does occur in the life cycle with regard to the type of tissue invaded by the sporozoite. In the subgenera which parasitize mammals (i.e. *Plasmodium, Laverania* and *Vinckeia*) only the liver parenchyma tissue is attacked. However, in the subgenera *Haemamoeba, Huffia, Giovannolaia* and *Novyella* of birds and *Carinia* and *Sauramoeba* of reptiles, the first cycle of schizogony, also referred to as the primary exoerythrocytic cycle, takes place in lymphoid-macrophage cells of the skin in the vicinity of the bite of the mosquito and the second and subsequent cycles of schizogony (secondary exoerythrocytic cycles) occur in lymphoid-macrophage cells in any location. In the malarial parasites of mammals, with the

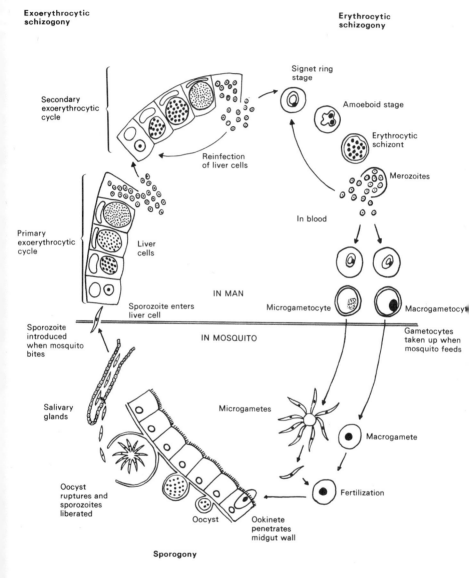

Figure 106 Life cycle of *Plasmodium vivax*.

exception of the subgenus *Laverania*, both primary and secondary exoerythrocytic schizogony cycles occur. In *Laverania* there is no secondary cycle.

Following exoerythrocytic schizogony the merozoites enter the blood-stream and penetrate red blood corpuscles, in which they commence a phase of growth. At this time a large vacuole appears in their structure to function both as a food vacuole and as a means of increasing their surface area. This is the so-called signet-ring stage. These forms feed and grow and are then known as trophozoites. Soon they become amoeboid prior to undergoing a cycle of multiplication (erythrocytic schizogony) when they produce a new generation of merozoites. Some of these merozoites develop into gametocytes, which are sexual stages. The gametocytes remain dormant, usually within the red blood corpuscles, although they may sometimes escape from the erythrocyte and are found in the plasma. Here they remain until either they are ingested by a mosquito of the appropriate species or they perish. Yet other merozoites reinvade erythrocytes to produce more schizonts. It is now thought that it is the release of the merozoites together with their stored excretory products which produces the fevers associated with malaria.

When a mosquito imbibes corpuscles containing gametocytes the cell walls are digested in the midgut and the parasites liberated. Some of the gametocytes, the macrogametocytes, become spherical and are then known as macrogametes, or female gametes. Others, the microgametocytes, undergo three nuclear divisions to produce eight nuclei, each of which is surrounded by a small amount of cytoplasm which develops a flagellum (exflagellation). These soon break free and are the flagellated microgametes. If one of these contacts a macrogamete fertilization occurs. The stimulus for gamete formation in the midgut of the mosquito is most likely the drop in temperature experienced on transference from the vertebrate to the arthropod host.

The zygote which is produced as a result of fertilization is motile and is called an ookinete. Like the sporozoite, this stage possesses organelles of penetration and locomotion and it passes through the peritrophic membrane lining the midgut and then digests its way through the single cell layer of the mosquito midgut wall to lie between the cell and the basement membrane. The ookinete secretes a thin cyst wall to become an oocyst and undergoes repeated nuclear division to produce numerous sporozoites. This process is similar to schizogony but as the end products are sporozoites and not merozoites it is known as sporogony. The first post-zygotic division, that is the first division of sporogony, is meiotic and thus the sporozoites are haploid. Indeed, it is only the zygote (ookinete) which is diploid, a phenomenon which is characteristic of the Sporozoa.

Eventually the oocyst wall and the basement membrane rupture to liberate the sporozoites into the haemocoel of the mosquito. These swim in the haemocoelic fluid and eventually, if successful, they reach the salivary glands, which they penetrate, and enter the lumen. When the mosquito feeds again it introduces some of these sporozoites into its new host together with saliva and, if the host is susceptible, the cycle recommences.

Human malaria

Four species of the genus *Plasmodium* may parasitize man, all of which produce clinical symptoms. These species are discussed below and their characteristics are given in Table 4.

1 *Plasmodium (Plasmodium) vivax*   This parasite gains its specific name from the fact that the amoeboid trophozoite stage is very active or lively. Once common in southern England this organism causes a recurring fever at forty-eight hour intervals, coincident with the release of merozoites at the completion of erythrocytic schizogony. Unfortunately this type of malaria is termed 'tertian malaria', which suggests a three-day fever cycle, but actually the terminology was coined to describe fever occurring on day one and next on day three, that is with a two-day periodicity. As this terminology is accepted by the medical profession it should be adhered to by zoologists to avoid even greater confusion.

Malaria caused by *Plasmodium vivax* is described as benign, for

Table 4 Human malarial parasites

Species of Plasmodium	Geographical location	Disease produced	Duration of exoerythro-cytic schizogony (days)	Duration of erythrocytic schizogony (days)	Duration of sporogony at 24°C (days)	Effect on host erythrocyte	
						Size	Cytoplasmic stippling
vivax	all tropical, subtropical and warm temperate regions	benign tertian malaria	8	2	9	enlarged	present—called Schüffner's dots
malariae	scattered throughout tropics and subtropics	benign quartan malaria	15	3	21	un-changed	normally absent but prolonged staining produces Ziemann's dots
ovale	tropical Africa and various other tropical and subtropical lands	benign ovale tertian malaria	9	2	16	enlarged	present—called Schüffner's dots
falciparum	all tropical, subtropical and warm temperate regions	malignant tertian malaria	6	2	11	un-changed	few large dots or streaks present—called Maurer's clefts

it is not a fatal disease although it does cause debilitation. The parasite may persist for several years in untreated cases, with a reservoir of infection remaining in the liver parenchyma cells. *P. vivax* produces enlargement of the host corpuscle, while stippling of the cytoplasm known as Schüffner's dots, which are probably of similar origin to those of *P. falciparum* (see later), is revealed on staining with Giemsa's stain (Fig. 107). It is not known why the corpuscle should become enlarged, for this cannot be explained as being due to pressure of the parasite on the corpuscle wall.

P. vivax is transmitted by many species of *Anopheles*, for example *A. stephensi, A. barbirostris, A. maculipennis* and *A. darlingi.*

2 *P. (P) malariae*   This malarial parasite produces a quartan disease in man, with erythrocytic schizogony cycles and hence fever every seventy-two hours, that is on day one and then next on day four. In common with *P. vivax* malaria this disease is also benign. The red blood corpuscles are not enlarged in *P. malariae* infections and with normal staining procedures no stippling is seen.

It is strange that no good vector of this parasite has been discovered, although development of small numbers of individuals will take place in a wide range of *Anopheles* species. In nature *A. gambiae, A. funestus* and *A. darlingi* have been found to be infected.

3 *P. (P) ovale*   This is the least common of the malarial parasites of man and produces a benign tertian disease. As in the case of *P. vivax* the host corpuscle exhibits stippling (Schüffner's dots) and is enlarged. Also, the host corpuscle becomes ovoid in prepared slides (hence the specific name of the parasite) and often ruptures, probably owing to fragility as a consequence of the infection.

A natural vector of *P. ovale* has never been identified positively, although in tropical Africa the *Anopheles* species *A. gambiae* and *A. funestus* are almost certainly the transmitters.

4 *P. (Laverania) falciparum*   This organism, which derives its specific name from the crescentic shape of its gametocytes, is both the most common and the most pathogenic of the human malarial parasites, producing a malignant tertian disease. It is peculiar in that it has no secondary exoerythrocytic cycle in its life history and that only young trophozoites (signet-ring stages) and mature gametocytes are seen in the peripheral blood (and hence blood films prepared from surface punctures). The intermediate forms are

found only in the blood vessels of deeper organs, but the reason for this is not clear. It has, however, been suggested that the infected corpuscles are more adhesive than uninfected ones and so stick to capillary walls, thus becoming entrapped in these sites.

The corpuscle containing this parasite is not enlarged but its cytoplasm contains stipples called Maurer's clefts. Studies using the electron microscope have revealed that these stipplings are fragments of membrane which have been cast from the parasite.

A wide range of *Anopheles* species may act as vectors for *P. falciparum*, among the more important ones being *A. funestus*, *A. gambiae*, *A. bancrofti* and *A. stephensi*.

Malaria of mammals other than man

Within the Mammalia the genus *Plasmodium* occurs in man, monkeys and African rats only. The two rat species, which can be transferred to laboratory rodents, are *P. (Vinckeia) berghei* and *P. (V) vinckei*, both of which are transmitted by the mosquito *Anopheles dureni*. Among the important species occurring in primates other than man are the following.

1 *P. (P) cynomolgi*   This is a parasite similar to *P. vivax*, which occurs in monkeys in India, Ceylon and the Far East and which has a tertian cycle. It is transmitted by various forest-dwelling *Anopheles* species (e.g. *A. hackeri*).

2 *P. (P) knowlesi*   This species is also parasitic in Asian monkeys but shows a quotidian (twenty-four hour) cycle. Like *P. cynomolgi* it is transmitted by *A. hackeri*.

3 *P. (P) cynomolgi bastianellii*   This parasite of monkeys (and man under experimental conditions) has a tertian cycle and is transmitted by *A. stephensi*.

Until recently *P. rodhaini* of chimpanzees was considered to be a distinct species but this has now been shown to be identical to *P. malariae* of man.

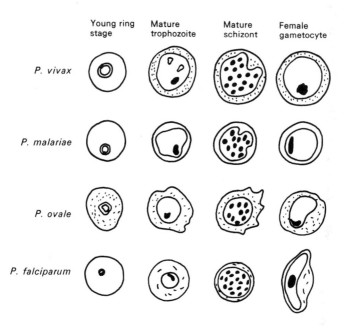

	Young ring stage	Mature trophozoite	Mature schizont	Female gametocyte
P. vivax				
P. malariae				
P. ovale				
P. falciparum				

Figure 107 Selected erythrocytic stages of human malarial parasites.

Important non-mammalian species

Only three species will be mentioned here, all of which belong to the subgenus *Haemamoeba*. These are *P.* (*H*) *gallinaceum*, primarily a parasite of the jungle fowl in Asia, but to which chickens are particularly susceptible; *P.* (*H*) *cathemerium* of passerine birds (e.g. sparrows), with a worldwide distribution; and *P.* (*H*) *relictum*, again ubiquitous, and parasitic in pigeons, ducks and passerines. The natural vector of *P. cathemerium* is unknown but in the laboratory it will develop in *Culex pipiens* and *C. pipiens fatigans*, while vectors of *P. gallinaceum* and *P. relictum* are *Mansonia crassipes* and *Culex pipiens fatigans* respectively.

Species also occur in reptiles and perhaps amphibians, but nothing is confirmed with regard to their mode of transmission.

Infections of man

In a primary infection of malaria the parasite undergoes one

(*P. falciparum*) or two exoerythrocytic cycles before entering the blood some six to fifteen days after infection. However, it is not until the number of parasites in the blood has built up to about 200 per mm^3 that symptoms appear at the end of erythrocytic schizogony. The attacks or paroxysms in the form of chills and fevers so characteristic of malaria occur at daily intervals at first and then typically every two or three days, depending on the species of malarial parasite. In subsequent invasions the two- or three-day paroxysms are apparent from the start of the infection. Each malarial attack begins with a chill which is accompanied by shivering, even though the body temperature is increased. A fever with headache, nausea and high temperature (often 41°C or more) follows the chill, after which there is a period of profuse sweating and finally a drop in body temperature to below 37°C. The body temperature then reverts to normal and remains so until the next attack.

In *P. vivax* infections the paroxysms occur every forty-eight hours for a period of from eight to fourteen days, after which time the patient recovers with a return to normal body temperature and a reduction in the parasitaemia. Relapses take place after a latent period of about a year or more and may persist for many years before they finally terminate.

P. ovale infections follow a similar pattern except that the patient is not subject to relapse, and *P. malariae* invasion is characterized by attacks at three-day intervals which are more mild and of shorter duration than those of *P. vivax* but which persist for a much longer time.

P. falciparum is the most virulent of the malarial parasites, with febrile attacks every two days which are less well defined than those of the other human malarial diseases. In fact, each attack may last for up to thirty-six hours and may have barely ended before the next begins. Paroxysms end after about ten days, when the body temperature returns to normal. However, a few days later a second series of attacks commences which may be more severe than the first. After some time this set of attacks disappears only to be replaced by more at about ten-day intervals for a duration of several months. Attacks finally become irregular and more mild and the

J

disease may terminate in from six to nine months, although
recrudescence may occur up to two years.

In addition to the sequence of attacks outlined above *P.
falciparum* infections are accompanied by circulatory malfunctions,
for erythrocytes adhere to one another and so obstruct capillaries
and interfere with the flow of blood to vital organs. The denial of
oxygen to the brain together with the effects of toxic excretions
produced by the parasites may give rise to loss of consciousness
and strokes, a condition referred to as 'cerebral malaria'. In addition,
gastro-intestinal malfunctions, heart failure and pneumonia are
common, as is the condition known as 'blackwater fever', which is
due to intravascular destruction of red corpuscles and the
subsequent release of haemoglobin in the urine.

It must be appreciated that in countries where malaria is
endemic reinfection is often continuous and hence the clinical
picture may appear complicated. Infected persons often show few
symptoms and may act as carriers (reservoirs) of the disease. Many
drugs have been employed to combat malaria, the more important
of these being *camoquine dihydrochloride* (*amodiaquine*),
daraprim (*pyrimethamine*), *chloroquine phosphate*, *paludrine*
(*proguanil hydrochloride*) and *primaquine*, which are all synthetic
drugs and normally replace the once commonly used natural
compound, quinine, an extract from the bark of the cinchona tree.
However, intravenous injections of quinine are still employed in
treating acute attacks of *P. falciparum* malaria.

Filariasis
Mosquitoes are the proven vectors of several species of filarial
nematodes, among those of greatest importance being *Wuchereria
bancrofti* and its variant *W. bancrofti* var. *pacifica*, *Brugia malayi*,
Dirofilaria immitis and *Setaria equina*.

In general, the life cycles of all of these parasites are similar. In
Wuchereria bancrofti, for example, the adults are located in the
lymphatic system of man where pair formation occurs, the two
worms remaining together after mating. Within the uterus of the

female worm the young nematodes, called microfilariae, develop and when fully formed are liberated into the lymph-stream from which they migrate into the blood. The microfilariae possess an extremely interesting distribution pattern in that they spend the daytime in the capillaries of the lungs and move to the peripheral circulation at night. This is, of course, an adaptation to enhance their chances of being transferred to a new host by a mosquito which bites at night, the microfilariae returning to the lungs by day for here food and oxygen are plentiful. When a mosquito feeds it imbibes microfilariae which are still enveloped by a sheath, thought to be equivalent to an egg membrane. It is, therefore, debatable whether or not the method of reproduction represents true viviparity, for the microfilariae may be classed not as larvae but as motile embryos.

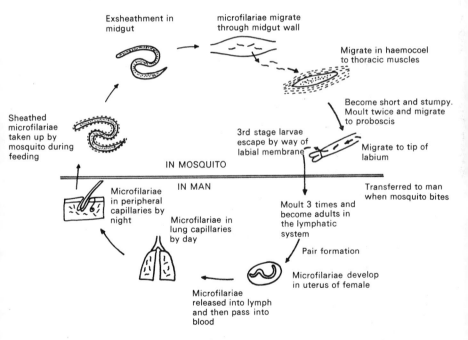

Figure 108 Life cycle of *Wuchereria bancrofti.*

Within the midgut of the mosquito the sheaths surrounding the microfilariae are ruptured, and they migrate through the midgut wall using piercing stylets to effect their penetration. Once through the gut wall the microfilariae are within the insect's haemocoel, and they migrate in the haemocoelic fluid to the thoracic musculature where they become short and stumpy and moult twice before re-entering the haemocoel to swim towards the mouthparts of the insect. When the mosquito next feeds the worms escape from its labium by breaking through the labial membrane (Fig. 108), the stimulus for their escape being the warmth of the skin adjacent to the mosquito's mouthparts. The juvenile worms wriggle on to the skin of the host which they penetrate either by way of the lesion produced by the insect's mouthparts or through intact skin using their own powers of penetration. They enter the peripheral circulation and, eventually, pass through the wall of a blood vessel

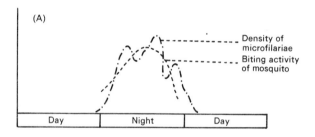

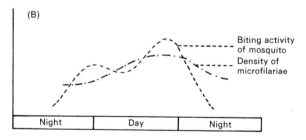

Figure 109 The microfilarial periodicity and biting activity of the vector plotted against time for A, *Wuchereria bancrofti* and *Culex pipiens fatigans* and B, *W. bancrofti* var. *pacifica* and *Aedes scutellaris polynesiensis*.

into the lymphatic system, where they undergo further moults to reach the adult stage some three months to a year later.

In *W. bancrofti* the peak in microfilarial swarming in the peripheral blood occurs between 2200 h and 0200 h; this can be correlated directly with the biting activity of the mosquito vector, for example *Culex pipiens fatigans* (Fig. 109 A). It is thought that the microfilarial activity is a direct consequence of the circadian rhythm of the host animal, for when a person changes his routine and remains awake at night and sleeps by day after some time the periodicity of microfilarial activity is also reversed.

W. bancrofti is distributed throughout the tropics (Fig. 110). Among the important vectors are *Culex pipiens fatigans*, *Anopheles barbirostris*, *Mansonia uniformis* and *Anopheles stephensi* in Asia; *Culex pipiens fatigans*, *Anopheles gambiae* and *Anopheles funestus* in Africa; and *Culex pipiens fatigans* and *Aedes aegypti* in the Americas and West Indies.

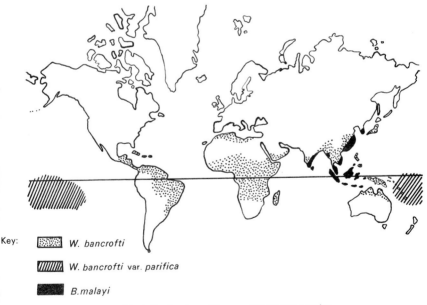

Key:

- W. bancrofti
- W. bancrofti var. parifica
- B. malayi

Figure 110 Geographical distribution of human filarial nematodes.

In contrast to *W. bancrofti* the variety *W. bancrofti* var. *pacifica* is described as subperiodic. The microfilariae of this nematode are identical to those of *W. bancrofti* although the adults are slightly smaller and differ in a few minor morphological details. The main difference concerns the periodicity of the microfilariae, which is slight, as indicated in Fig. 109 B. Development of *W. bancrofti* var. *pacifica* occurs in mosquitoes indigenous to the South Pacific Islands, for example *Aedes scutellaris polynesiensis* and *A. s. pseudoscutellaris*. These mosquitoes are peculiar in that they feed by day, which is thought to account for the change in periodicity of this filarial worm.

Yet a third filarial worm which affects man occurs in Indonesia, Malaysia, China, Japan, India and Ceylon. This is *Brugia malayi*, of which two forms have been recognized: the *nocturnal periodic form*, found on the west coast of the Malay peninsula and in the other countries listed above, which is transmitted by various *Anopheles* and *Mansonia* species, for example *A. barbirostris* and *M. longipalpis*, and is a parasite of man only; and the *semi-nocturnal form*, occurring on the east coast of Malaysia only, which, although transmissible to man, is primarily a parasite of monkeys and so is an example of a zoonosis, and is transmitted by *Mansonia annulata* and *M. uniformis*.

Two filarial worms affecting domesticated animals now deserve mention. They are *Dirofilaria immitis*, a parasite of the dog, cat, fox and wolf, and *Setaria equina*, found in various equines.

Adult *Dirofilaria immitis* live mainly in the right ventricle and pulmonary artery, although they do parasitize other parts of the body. The female releases microfilariae directly into the bloodstream and once again a migration takes place between peripheral and deeper vessels, although the pattern of movement varies in different parts of the world. Thus the peak in numbers in the peripheral blood is at about 1600 to 1700 h in North America and about 1800 h in Asia. The life history of *D. immitis* is essentially similar to that of *Wuchereria bancrofti* but with several important differences. Thus after entering the midgut of the mosquito the microfilariae migrate posteriorly to enter the Malpighian tubules.

Here they penetrate tubule cells and remain in this location for about two weeks. Within the cells they become short, stumpy second-stage larvae which emerge and pass within the haemocoel to the labium of the insect, where they moult to become infective third-stage larvae. *D. immitis* is transmitted by many *Culex, Aedes, Anopheles* and *Myzorhynchus* species, for example *Anopheles quadrimaculatus* in North America.

   Setaria equina is parasitic as an adult in the peritoneal cavity and scrotum of equines in all parts of the world. Microfilariae are liberated and swarm in the peripheral blood in the evening, from which site they are abstracted by one of a number of culicine mosquitoes, such as *Aedes aegypti*. In all important respects the life cycle of this non-pathogenic worm is identical to that of *Wuchereria bancrofti.*

Infections of man and domesticated animals
1 *Filariasis in man*   The condition of gross enlargement of body components produced by the obstruction of lymphatic channels by adult worms and developing microfilariae is called elephantiasis. The worms may either physically block lymphatic ducts or may cause inflammatory thickenings of the vessel walls and so lead to obstruction indirectly. It is sometimes found that worms become calcified due to host reaction and so form a permanent blockage of the lymphatic system. The fully developed microfilariae in the blood-stream appear to produce no harmful effects.

   Elephantiasis is not fully explained by the statement that lymphatic vessels become obstructed. Actually, when a duct is blocked, new, compensatory routes are formed with a result that these newly formed circulations are used excessively and, together with parasitized vessels up to the region of obstruction, become dilated. This increase in diameter is transmitted to the surrounding tissues and so the affected region of the body becomes swollen.

   Body enlargement due to parasitic invasion is caused not only by the mosquito-borne *Wuchereria bancrofti, W. bancrofti* var. *pacifica* and *Brugia malayi* but also by *Onchocerca volvulus* transmitted by *Simulium* (see page 180) and *Loa loa* which is disseminated by

Chrysops (see page 178). As far as the mosquito-borne worms are concerned, the pathological effects of *W. bancrofti* and *B. malayi* are essentially similar, whereas those produced by *W. bancrofti* var. *pacifica* are often more severe and more extensive.

There is no really satisfactory chemotherapeutic treatment for human filariasis at present. Administration of *hetrazan* (*diethyl carbamazine*) kills the microfilariae, but this is, of course, a method of control only in that it is denying the mosquito the microfilariae when it feeds. It does not help the patient. The treatment available ls to either excise affected tissues or to irradicate them with X-rays accompanied by massage and the use of elasticated supports.

2 *Filariasis in dogs* Adults of *Dirofilaria immitis* inhabit the circulatory system, in particular the heart and adjacent vessels, and although in many cases their presence may cause no appreciable symptoms they may give rise to cardiac stress and insufficiency, for example lack of stamina and increased rate of breathing. *Hetrazan* is effective in controlling both microfilariae and adults in dogs.

Virus diseases
A large number of virus diseases are transmitted by mosquitoes, some of the more important ones being listed in Table 5. Of these, two deserve special mention here, yellow fever and dengue, both of

Table 5 Important mosquito-borne virus diseases of man

Virus and main symptoms	Geographical distribution	Main vectors
GROUP A VIRUSES		
Eastern equine encephalomyelitis (attacks nervous system; fever)	Eastern USA and South America	*Culiseta melanura* and various *Aedes* and *Culex* species

Virus and main symptoms	Geographical distribution	Main vectors
Western equine encephalomyelitis (attacks nervous system; like dengue)	Western USA, South America and Central Europe	Culex tarsalis
Venezuelan equine encephalomyelitis (attacks nervous system; fever)	Caribbean and South America	Culex pipiens fatigans and Aedes serratus
Chikungunya (like dengue)	East and South Africa	Aedes africanus and Aedes aegypti
Mayaro (fever)	West Indies and South America	Mansonia venezuelensis
Semliki Forest (attacks nervous system)	East and West Africa	Aedes abnormalis
Sindbis (attacks nervous system)	North and South Africa, India and Malaya	Culex univittatus
O'nyong-nyong (like dengue)	East and West Africa	Anopheles funestus
Middleburg (attacks nervous system; fever)	South Africa	Aedes caballus
Uruma (attacks viscera; fever)	South America	?

GROUP B VIRUSES

| Dengue I (see text) | East and South Asia (coastal) and South West Pacific | Aedes albopictus and Aedes aegypti |

[continued]

Virus and main symptoms	Geographical distribution	Main vectors
Dengue II (see text)	India, West Indies, New Guinea and Thailand	*Aedes scutellaris* complex and *Aedes aegypti*
Dengue III and IV (see text)	Philippines	*Aedes albopictus* and *Aedes aegypti*
Japanese B (attacks nervous system; fever)	Far East, India and South West Pacific	*Culex pipiens pallens*
St Louis (attacks nervous system)	USA, West Indies and Central and South America	*Culex pipiens* complex
West Nile (like dengue)	Africa, Middle East and India	*Culex molestus*
Uganda S (no symptoms in man)	East and West Africa, India and Far East	*Aedes aegypti*
Ilheus (attacks nervous system)	South America and West Indies	*Aedes aegypti* and *Sabethes chloropictus*
Spondweni (attacks nervous system)	South Africa and Nigeria	*Aedes vigilax*
Wesselsbron (fever; like influenza)	South Africa	*Aedes caballus* and *Aedes circumluteolus*
Zika Forest (attacks nervous system and viscera)	East and West Africa	*Aedes africanus*
Yellow fever (see text)	Africa and South America	*Aedes aegypti*

Virus and main symptoms	Geographical distribution	Main vectors
Murray Valley encephalitis (attacks nervous system; fever)	Australia and New Guinea	Aedes scutellaris complex and Culex tarsalis
GROUP C VIRUSES		
Marituba (attacks nervous system)	Brazil	various Aedes and Culex species
Oriboea (attacks nervous system)	Brazil	various Aedes and Culex species
BUNYAMWERA GROUP		
Bunyamwera (attacks nervous system; fever)	East, West and South Africa	various Aedes species
UNGROUPED VIRUSES		
Rift Valley fever (attacks viscera; fever)	East, Central and South Africa	Aedes tarsalis and Aedes africanus

which cause serious debility in man, the former commonly terminating in death in untreated cases.

Yellow fever
The distribution of yellow fever is much wider than was formerly supposed. Recent immunological surveys have shown that it is endemic in much of Africa and Central South America. Until quite recently the virus was widely distributed in the West Indies and

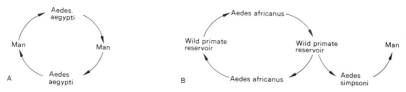

Figure 111 Transmission pattern of yellow fever. (For further explanation see text.)

North America, with outbreaks in Europe reported on numerous occasions.

From intensive studies on the epidemiology of yellow fever it has become apparent that there are two types of fever. The first of these is the 'urban or rural' variety and is a human disease associated with human habitations. In both Africa and America the insect vector is *Aedes aegypti* and transmission is solely between this mosquito and man (Fig. 111 A).

The second type of the disease is the 'jungle or sylvatic' yellow fever which affects both man and wild animals, the latter acting as sylvan reservoir hosts. Among the animals which have been incriminated as reservoir hosts are various monkeys, marmosets, anteaters, opossums, armadillos, sloths, capybara and mice. The major vectors of this variant of the fever are *Aedes simpsoni*, *A. africanus* and *Mansonia africana* in Africa and *Haemagogus spegazzinii*, *H. s. falco*, *Aedes fluviatilis* and *Sabethes chloropterus* in America. All of these are day-biting insects and transmit the disease from, say, monkeys to man in plantations and forest clearings. Some mosquitoes feed mainly on man and are referred to as being anthropophilic, whereas others show preference for non-human hosts (zoophilic insects). Hence it is likely that more than one species of mosquito is responsible for the cycling of jungle yellow fever between sylvan and human hosts, as is indicated in Fig. 111 B.

Yellow fever virus is a filterable ultravirus which, when taken up from the blood of an infected animal, passes through the gut wall to become distributed throughout the body of the insect. Multiplication of the virus takes place for between four and eighteen days, depending on the ambient temperature, and at the end of this time the virus particles have reached the salivary glands and are transferred to a new host when the mosquito salivates during the feeding process. It is also possible to transmit the virus by swallowing the infected mosquitoes and by crushing them on to the body surface, the virus particles being capable of penetrating unbroken human skin.

Once a mosquito becomes infected it remains so for the rest of its life, but there is no evidence to suggest that either trans-ovarial or trans-stadial transmission occur. In addition to mosquitoes, it has been shown that yellow fever virus can be disseminated by ticks (*Amblyomma* and *Ornithodorus* species), by bugs (*Panstrongylus* species), by fleas (*Ctenocephalides* species) and by flies (*Stomoxys* species).

The symptoms of yellow fever range from being very mild to extremely severe. In the former case they take the form of fever and headaches which last for some two or three days. However, more usually, the three to six day incubation period is followed by symptoms of high fever for three or four days, after which there is a return to normal body temperature for about four days when the skin and sclerotic coats of the eyes become yellow. This symptom, which gives the disease its name, results from the virus attacking the liver, producing necrosis and jaundice. The third and final stage of the disease produces headaches, muscular pain, and aches in the bones and the stomach region. Spontaneous haemorrhages may also commence and the disease is often fatal.

No specific treatment for this disease exists and recovery is dependent on careful nursing and the relief of vomiting, aches and insomnia. Vaccination to prevent development of the disease is highly successful and produces yellow fever antibodies in the blood after about two weeks which persist for several years.

Dengue (breakbone fever)

Found in tropical and subtropical lands, dengue is caused by a filterable virus which exists in at least four immunologically distinct but antigenically related strains. As with yellow fever the virus multiplies in the tissues of the mosquito and can be detected throughout its body. Transmission occurs on salivation, and the insect, once infected, remains so for life. Congenital transmission has not been demonstrated.

The main vector of dengue is *Aedes aegypti*. This is aided by *Aedes albopictus* in the Philippines, Japan, Sumatra and Hawaii; *Aedes scutellaris polynesiensis* in the Pacific; *A. s. hebrideus* in New Guinea; and *A. obturbans* in Formosa. Like yellow fever it is believed that dengue exists as both urban and jungle types, the latter being a zoonosis with monkeys acting as reservoirs of infection.

Dengue is, without doubt, the most painful of all fevers. Following the five to nine day incubation period there are symptoms of aches in the muscles and joints, headaches and fever which last for two or three days. This phase of the illness is replaced by a period of one to three days duration when there is a return to both normal body temperature and good health. But the fever soon returns, together with pains and a rash which covers most of the body apart from the face. Although dengue is the cause of debility it is rarely fatal. No specific treatment is recommended except for rest and the relief of pain.

Other diseases

It is likely that mosquitoes will be shown to be disseminators of many bacterial and related organisms although at present only a few such diseases are known to be so transmitted. Among these are *Treponema pertenue*, a spirochaete producing a contagious condition in man called yaws (frambesia) in North and South America, and *Brucella* (=*Pasteurella*) *tularensis*, the bacterium responsible for tularaemia in man and other animals in America, Europe, Asia and North Africa. Both of these organisms are carried by *Aedes aegypti*, although mosquitoes do not provide the only means of transmission.

In many parts of Central and South America certain species of the mosquito genus *Psorophora* have been shown to transport eggs of the bot fly, *Dermatobia hominis*. In Central America the mosquito vector is *Psorophora lutzii*, while in South America other species of this genus are involved, for example *P. ferox* in Columbia.

9
Leishmaniasis and other sandfly-borne diseases

Three diseases of man are known to be transmitted by sandflies: leishmaniasis, oroya fever and papataci fever. The first of these is a protozoan disease and exists in several forms which are differentiated, in the main, on the region of the body which they invade. Broadly speaking, kala-azar is leishmaniasis of the visceral organs; oriental sore is the disease involving the skin; and espundia is mucocutaneous leishmaniasis, affecting the skin and sometimes the mucous membranes. Of the remaining two sandfly-transmitted diseases, oroya fever is caused by a bacillus-like organism and papataci fever by a virus.

Leishmaniasis
Leishmaniasis is the collective name given to the diseases of man caused by members of the genus *Leishmania*. It is of interest that although there are a number of important leishmanias which infect man there is none parasitic in domesticated animals, although in some areas dogs in particular act as reservoirs for the human disease.

Characteristically, members of the genus *Leishmania* frequent the lymphoid-macrophage cells of vertebrates in a morphological form called the amastigote, or Leishman–Donovan body, and the midgut and foregut regions of sandflies as forms called promastigotes (Fig. 112). For a full description of these morphological stages, which are found throughout the protozoan order Kinetoplastida, reference should be made to chapter 10.

Species of leishmanias
Members of the genus *Leishmania* have been reported from

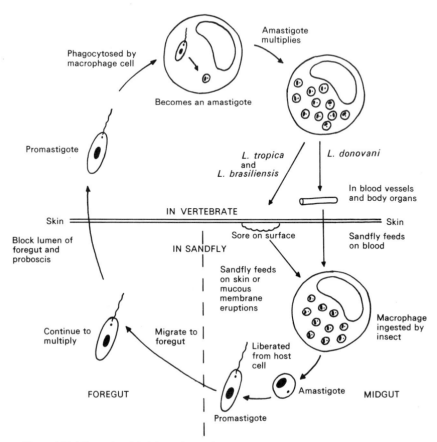

Figure 112 Life cycle of *Leishmania* species.

mammals and from lizards. At the present time about ten species have been described from reptiles and it is of interest that some of these show an evolutionary sequence ranging from gut parasites to blood parasites transmitted by an insect vector. About half of the species in lizards occur in the gut, for example *L. chameleonis*, restricted to the cloaca of chameleons, which is transferred when faeces containing leishmanias are expelled from one host and ingested by another.

L. henrici was discovered in lizards of the genus *Anolis* in

Martinique, and although it is found in the intestine it can invade the blood-stream where it survives without difficulty. The remaining species of *Leishmania* found in lizards are blood and tissue forms, one such species being *L. adleri* from *Latastia* species in Kenya. For their perpetuation all blood parasites require a haematophagous vector and in the case of *L. adleri* it is the sandfly, *Phlebotomus clydei*.

In members of the class Mammalia leishmanias produce obvious diseases in man only with dogs, foxes, monkeys, gerbils, squirrels, rats, mice and possibly other animals acting as reservoirs for the human diseases. Thus human leishmaniasis, with the possible exception of kala-azar caused by *L. donovani* in India and East Africa, is a zoonosis with the animal reservoirs, often domestic dogs, being a source of human infection (Fig. 113).

It is usual to recognize three principal species of *Leishmania* parasitic in man, namely *L. donovani*, *L. tropica* and *L. brasiliensis* (Table 6). All species of *Leishmania*, with the notable exception of *L. enriettii*, a parasite of guinea-pigs in South America, are morphologically similar and can be differentiated only by their pathological manifestations, peculiarities of physiology and life history, and their geographical distribution. In *L. enriettii* the amastigote stage is large (6 μm $\times$ 3 μm) and ovoid, whereas in the remaining species the amastigotes are more circular in outline and measure between 2 and 4 μm in diameter.

Returning to the human leishmanias, it was found to be possible to subdivide the three species on the clinical picture which they produce, their pathogenicity and their response to treatment. It is still valid to retain the three species for, as with all protozoan infections, a single species need not necessarily give a

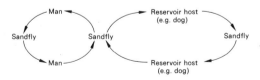

Figure 113 Transmission pattern of human leishmaniasis.

uniform picture. However, separation at the subspecies level has
been attempted, in particular in the case of *L. brasiliensis*, where
five subspecies have been designated: *L. b. brasiliensis*, *L. b.
guyanensis*, *L. b. mexicana*, *L. b. peruviana* and *L. b. pifanoi*. The
nature of the diseases produced, their geographical distribution, and
major hosts and important reservoirs of the causative agents are
given in Table 6. Subspecific classification has not been attempted
in the case of *L. donovani* although differences in the disease occur
throughout its geographical range in respect of vectors, reservoir
hosts and susceptibility of man (Table 6). With regard to the last
point, the parasite in the Mediterranean region and North Africa
affects young children only, due to the production of antibodies in
children over the age of about six which destroys the protozoans.
This has led to the use of the name *Leishmania donovani* var.
infantum to describe this parasite, but its adoption is neither
justified nor advisable.

In Indian and East African kala-azar a condition of post kala-
azar dermal leishmaniasis may occur, affecting areas of the skin

Table 6 Details of leishmanial parasites of man

Species of Leishmania	Disease produced	Geographical distribution	Major vectors	Important reservoirs	Remarks on taxonomy
L. donovani	visceral leishmaniasis or kala-azar (in marco-phages in liver, bone marrow, lymph nodes and blood)	India	*P. argentipes*	—	
		China	*P. chinensis* *P. sergenti*	dog	
		Mediter-ranean region and North Africa	*P. perniciosus* *P. major*	dog	often called *L. donovani* var. *infantum*
		East Africa	*P. orientalis* *P. martini*	monkeys, gerbils and ground squirrels	
		Middle East and Russia	*P. papatasii*	dog	
		South America	*P. intermedius* *P. longipalpis*	dog and fox	

Species of Leishmania	Disease produced	Geographical distribution	Major vectors	Important reservoirs	Remarks on taxonomy
L. tropica	cutaneous leishmaniasis or oriental sore (in macrophages in skin and subcutaneous tissues and adjacent lymph nodes)	Mediterranean region North, Central and West Africa, Middle and Far East and India Central Asia	P. sergenti P. papatasii P. caucasicus	 dog, gerbils and other wild rodents	produce dry sores—urban leishmaniasis (L. tropica minor)—and wet sores—rural leishmaniasis (L. tropica major)
L. brasiliensis	espundia— malignant, with metastatic invasion of mucosa and skin	Brazil	P. intermedius P. migonei P. whitmani	dog and paca	often called L. b. brasiliensis
	benign, with nasal mucosa sometimes involved as well as skin	French Guinea, Costa Rica and Panama	P. evansi P. migonei	rats	often called L. b. guyanensis
	benign, with no invasion of mucosa but with weeping ulcerations	Mexico, Honduras and Guatemala	P. cruciatus P. panamensis P. longipalpis	rats and mice	often called L. b. mexicana
	benign, with no invasion of mucosa but with dry ulcerations	Peru, Bolivia and Ecuador	P. noguchi P. verrucarum	dog	often called L. b. peruviana
	malignant, with no invasion of mucosa but with extensive cutaneous lesions	Venezuela and Amazon region	P. panamensis	unknown	often called L. b. pifanoi

long after cure of the visceral disease. Such skin regions contain
Leishman–Donovan bodies in infected macrophages, and these are
accessible to sandflies when feeding on the skin. Man thus fills the
role of a reservoir of the disease in these geographical localities. It
is possible that wild rodents may also act as reservoir hosts in
India, but none has been proven at the present time; neither is it
known whether or not the main vector of kala-azar in India, namely
Phlebotomus argentipes, feeds on rodents. In East Africa wild
animals, for example cercopithecoid monkeys, gerbils and ground
squirrels, harbour the disease in jungles and man may incidentally
become infected if he ventures into such regions. However,
because of the involvement of the skin people may then be
responsible for passing the disease to others in human communities
where sandflies are present. The transmission pattern for kala-azar
in India and East Africa may be depicted as shown in Fig. 114.

Two types of sores (cutaneous leishmaniasis) can be recognized
in *L. tropica* infections, the wet sores found mainly in rural areas
and the dry sores which are normally urban. This has led to the
adoption by some authorities of two subspecies, namely *L. tropica
major* for the causal agent of the wet sore condition and *L. tropica
minor* for the aetiological agent responsible for dry sore
leishmaniasis (Table 6).

Life histories and transmission
Although information is not available for all species, it appears that
there is uniformity regarding the life cycles and methods of
transmission of leishmanias. The one major variation which does
occur concerns the sites within the body of the vertebrate in which

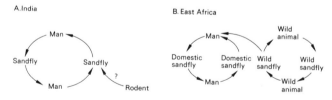

Figure 114 Transmission pattern of kala-azar in India (A) and East Africa (B).

the parasite is to be found, which in turn determines the mode of uptake of the protozoans by the vectors.

When an infected sandfly bites a susceptible mammal leishmanial parasites in the form of promastigotes are either deposited directly from the proboscis or regurgitated from the blocked gut into the lesion (Fig. 115). These forms are soon phagocytosed by macrophages in the skin, but instead of being destroyed by these cells the promastigotes survive and after becoming non-flagellated amastigotes they divide repeatedly every twenty-four hours or so until they occupy most of the space within the host cell membrane. These amastigotes are often referred to as Leishman—Donovan bodies after the names of their discoverers. The life of a macrophage is limited and when it dies it liberates the amastigotes which, presumably, are taken up by other phagocytic macrophage cells. During their restricted life span macrophages divide by binary fission, and it is believed that when this happens amastigotes are shared between the newly formed daughter cells.

In the case of *L. tropica* and *L. brasiliensis* the infected macrophages are normally restricted to the superficial tissues. In *L. donovani*, however, amastigotes migrate to deeper tissues, for example the liver, spleen, lymph nodes and bone marrow, and are

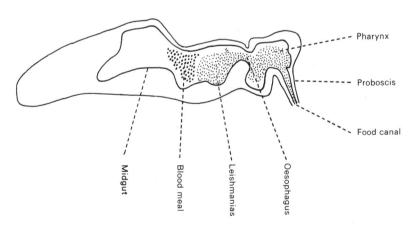

Figure 115 Longitudinal section through *Phlebotomus* showing leishmanias in gut.

also found in the circulating blood. In all of these situations they
become phagocytosed and multiply as indicated above.

Amastigotes of *L. tropica* are found in the skin and
subcutaneous tissues, and sometimes in adjacent lymph nodes.
Occasionally, eruptions of the skin occur producing ulcerations
containing infected macrophages. As there are no circulating
leishmanias the sandfly vector (e.g. *Phlebotomus papatasii*) must
feed directly from a surface ulcer in order to transmit the disease.
Similarly, in *L. brasiliensis* there are no forms in the blood, although
parasites are found in macrophages not only in the skin but also in
the mucous membranes of the mouth, nose and pharynx. Once
again the uptake of parasites by the vector (e.g. *Phlebotomus
intermedius*) is dependent on its feeding on skin eruptions.

In contrast to these two species, *L. donovani* occurs in various
visceral organs and in the circulating blood. Thus sandflies such as
Phlebotomus argentipes feeding on the blood of an infected person
would ingest parasitized macrophages and hence transmit the
disease.

A third method by which sandflies can become infected is
illustrated in the uptake of *L. donovani* in India and East Africa (see
above), where the skin of humans become uniformly infected with
macrophages containing Leishman–Donovan bodies after the main
disease is cured. Hence sandflies like *Phlebotomus argentipes*
become infected when feeding on unbroken skin. The same method
of transmission also occurs when flies feed on dogs naturally
infected with visceral leishmaniasis.

Within the vector the ingested macrophages are digested in the
midgut (Fig. 112), thus releasing the amastigotes which develop a
flagellum and undergo other changes to become promastigote
forms. This morphological change is probably adaptive in the same
way as it is in trypanosomes, and is perhaps similar in that a
mitochondrion is being proliferated in the invertebrate host with an
accompanied change in terminal respiration. Also, the flagellum is
functional in the insect host for the subsequent migrations and for
anchoring the protozoan to the wall of the insect's gut.

The promastigotes subsequently divide and continue to multiply as they move anteriorly into the foregut of the insect. As a result of their proliferation they completely fill the lumen of the foregut and proboscis such that when the sandfly attempts to feed some promastigotes are expelled into the wound produced by the insect's mouthparts as a regurgitation. The time taken for the parasite to complete its cycle in the sandfly varies with temperature, but, on average, takes about four or five days, which approximates to the periodicity of feeding of the vector.

Infections of man
1 *Visceral leishmaniasis, or kala-azar*   When introduced into man the promastigotes of *L. donovani* are taken up by macrophages at the site of the bite and there they multiply and later (as amastigotes) invade visceral organs, for example the spleen, liver and bone marrow. The parasite destroys the macrophages in the process and may produce a generalized infection of the reticulo-endothelial system of the body, giving lymph node and spleen enlargement, and anaemia.

The disease is usually fatal unless treated with antimony compounds, for example *pentostam* (*sodium stibo-gluconate*), which alleviate symptoms by killing the parasites. There is, however, evidence to suggest that in India in particular comparatively mild and self-terminating cases do occur.

2 *Cutaneous leishmaniasis, or oriental sore*   In this disease the promastigotes of *L. tropica*, which become phagocytosed by the skin macrophages, multiply and later invade other similar skin cells, producing lesions and ulcers which erupt on to the skin surface. These invariably heal, leaving a scar, and the disease is never fatal. Oriental sore is treated by administering either various trivalent and pentavalent antimony compounds or diamidines, for example *pentamidine* and *hydroxystilbamidine*.

3 *Mucocutaneous leishmaniasis, or espundia*   This disease is similar to oriental sore except that, following the establishment of sores in the skin, there is a metastatic invasion of the mucous

membranes which may involve the nasal septum, palate, mouth, pharynx, larynx and rarely the penis and vulva. Mucous membrane invasion results in eroding lesions and may lead to considerable deformity; for example the nose may be eroded away and, if the larynx is affected, the voice may be lost. Accompanying these symptoms are those of fever, anaemia, local pain and malaise.

The disease usually lasts for several years and normally terminates in death from complications like bronchopneumonia and septicemia rather than from the primary lesions themselves. Treatment is usually successful if administered before metastasis has involved the mucous membranes, in which case *cycloguanil pamoate* and the drugs used to combat cutaneous leishmaniasis may be employed. Once the mucous membranes have been infected the treatment may be prolonged with antimony compounds used to control the leishmanias and antibiotics to deal with secondary bacterial infection.

Oroya fever (bartonellosis, or Carrion's disease)

The aetiological agent of oroya fever is a bacillus-like organism of uncertain taxonomic position called *Bartonella bacilliformis*, found in parts of South America, notably Peru, Ecuador, Columbia, Chile, Bolivia and Guatemala. The proven mechanical transmitter of this disease is *Phlebotomus verrucarum*, although this is most probably aided by *P. noguchii, P. peruensis* and *P. columbianus*. It is possible that in the future an animal reservoir for oroya fever may be discovered, but at present there is no reason to regard it as being anything but a solely human disease.

Bartonella bacilliformis is found in the erythrocytes of man in times of fever and in the reticulo-endothelial cells of lymph nodes, the liver, the spleen and bone marrow at all times. Two types of the organism are seen in the red cells: rod-shaped forms measuring 2 μm × 0·5 μm and spherical forms about 1 μm in diameter (Fig. 116). The organism invades erythrocytes, multiplies and destroys the cells, rapidly giving rise to severe anaemia. As well as affecting blood cells the metabolic by-products liberated from the parasite destroy cells in the liver, spleen and other lymphatic organs.

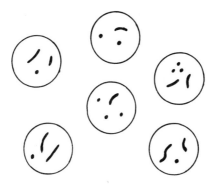

Figure 116 Bartonella bacilliformis in red blood corpuscles.

Accompanying the pathological picture outlined above are symptoms of malaise, low fever and pains in the head and limbs. The mortality rate is high, with about 40 per cent of infected cases terminating in death within two or three weeks of parasitic invasion. Treatment involves the administration of *chloramphenicol*, which prevents the risk of fulminating *Salmonella* infection, and the disease can be made less severe by giving prophylactic vaccinations. There is no evidence that any drug acts specifically on the *Bartonella* infection.

Sometimes local connective tissue invasion by *B. bacilliformis* may occur which is referred to as Verruga Peruana or localized bartonellosis. This gives skin lesions and is a condition which normally is seen in the wake of oroya fever some thirty to forty days after the disappearance of febrile symptoms. Occasionally, however, the initial fever may be lacking and the disease may commence with connective tissue invasion.

Papataci, or sandfly, fever
This virus disease is prevalent in the Mediterranean region and extends eastwards through to India, being transmitted by the bite of *Phlebotomus papatasii*. Both trans-ovarial and trans-stadial transmission have been demonstrated in this sandfly for adults die in November and are replaced by infective next-generation flies the

following April. The disease thus prevails between the months of
May to October. Sandfly fever is also reputed to occur in parts of
South America and the Caribbean, where it is probably transmitted
by several species of *Phlebotomus*, and is reported from China,
where the vectors are said to be *P. chinensis* and *P. mongolensis*.
Once infected, the sandflies remain so for life.

Papataci fever is caused by a filterable virus injected into man in
the saliva of the sandfly following a phase of multiplication in the
fly after the pattern shown by yellow fever virus in mosquitoes (see
page 126). For the first day or so after its introduction into man the
virus is found in the blood and only during this time can sandflies
take up the virus. A week after the parasite has entered man a
severe fever is experienced and, although there is no rash, the face
is flushed and swollen. Pains in the head, neck, back and legs
follow and then general muscular aches and drowsiness are
exhibited with the person remaining debilitated, particularly
mentally, for a further week or two. No complications of the disease
are seen and full recovery is virtually assured. There is at the
present time no successful prophylactic vaccine to combat sandfly
fever and the treatment of opium administration serves to relieve
symptoms rather than attack the virus.

10

Trypanosomiasis

Trypanosomiasis is the name given to the disease caused by species of the genus *Trypanosoma*. With the exception of *Trypanosoma evansi equiperdum*, a venereally transmitted disease of horses, these flagellates occur in a vertebrate host and are passed from one host to another by an invertebrate animal. In the case of trypanosomes of aquatic vertebrates (fish and amphibians) the disseminating invertebrates are leeches, whilst those of reptiles, birds and mammals are arthropods. Apart from members of the subgenus *Endotrypanum*, a parasite found within the red blood corpuscles of sloths in South America, trypanosomes are located in the blood plasma and within certain body tissues of the vertebrate host.

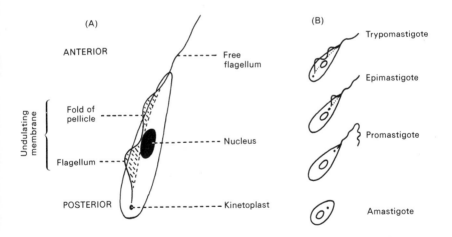

Figure 117 The major organelles of a trypanosome as seen using a light microscope (A) and the characteristics of the four forms which may be distinguished during the life cycle (B).

During its life cycle a trypanosome passes through a number of different morphological stages which are reflections of the changing physiological state of the parasite. The morphology of one of these stages, named the trypomastigote (=trypanosome) stage, is shown in Fig. 117 A. This is an elongated form in which the kinetoplast is placed posteriorly and which has a well-developed undulating membrane and a free flagellum. The other stages which exist are the epimastigote (crithidial) stage, an elongated form with the kinetoplast situated just anterior to the nucleus and with a small undulating membrane and a long free flagellum; the promastigote (leptomonad) stage, also elongated but with the kinetoplast located

Table 7 Characteristics of the major grouping of trypanosomes

Group	Subgenus	Position of nucleus	Kinetoplast Position	Size	Presence of free flagellum	Shape of posterior end
Lewisi group	Megatrypanum Herpetosoma Schizotrypanum	central or slightly anterior of central	aterminal	large	present	pointed
Vivax group	Duttonella	central	terminal	large	present	broadly rounded
Congolense group	Nannomonas	central	sub-terminal	medium	absent	broadly rounded
Brucei group	Pycnomonas	central	sub-terminal	small	present	pointed
	Trypanozoon		(absent in T. equinum)		(except in 'stumpy' forms of brucei sub-species)	narrowly rounded

at the anterior extremity; and the amastigote (leishmanial) stage, a form which differs from the others in that it is spherical and lacks both an undulating membrane and a free flagellum, although there is a conspicuous kinetoplast. All of these stages are shown in Fig. 117 B.

Subdivisions of the genus

Within the genus *Trypanosoma* a number of subdivisions have been devised to distinguish morphologically and physiologically differing forms. Some authors refer to the divisions as groups of no taxonomic status, while others allocate the varieties to the status of subgenera. The characteristics used to classify the flagellates are the position of the nucleus, the size and location of the kinetoplast, the presence or absence of a free flagellum and the shape of the posterior extremity. Table 7 gives a pictorial representation of members of the four groups as exemplified by *T. lewisi* (Lewisi group), *T. vivax vivax* (Vivax group), *T. congolense* (Congolense group) and *T. brucei brucei* (Brucei group). The Lewisi group may be equated with the subgenera *Megatrypanum*, *Herpetosoma* and *Schizotrypanum* and the Brucei group with the subgenera *Pycnomonas* and *Trypanozoon*. The Vivax and Congolense groups are the subgenera *Duttonella* and *Nannomonas* respectively of the alternative scheme.

Species of trypanosomes of non-mammalian vertebrates

There are numerous species of the genus *Trypanosoma* which are common parasites of fresh-water and marine fish, amphibians, reptiles and birds. Trypanosomes of non-mammalian hosts have received less attention than those affecting man and his domesticated stock, the best-known examples being the leech-transmitted *T. rotatorium* of the frog and *T. grayi* found in the crocodile and disseminated by the tsetse fly, *Glossina palpalis*.

Trypanosomes of mammals (Table 8)

As mentioned above, apart from *T. evansi equiperdum*, the causative agent of dourine of horses, all of the trypanosomes of

Table 8 Data on the main species of trypanosomes of mammals

Section	Subgenus	Species of Trypanosoma	Approx. length (μ m)	Geographical distribution
Salivaria (anterior station development)	Duttonella	T. vivax vivax	20–25	East, West and Central Africa
		T. v. viennei	20–25	Central and South America, Mauritius and West Indies
		T. uniforme	12–18	Uganda and Congo
	Nannomonas	T. congolense	10–20	East, West and Central Africa
		T. simiae	15–20	East, West, Central and parts of South Africa
	Pycnomonas	T. suis	13–18	Tanzania and Congo
	Trypanozoon	T. brucei brucei	15 (stumpy) to 30 (slender)	East, West, Central and parts of South Africa
		T. b. gambiense		West and Central Africa
		T. b. rhodesiense		East and Central Africa
		T. equinum	20–30	South America
		T. evansi evansi	20–30	Asia, Far East, North Africa, Mauritius, Central and South America
		T. evansi equiperdum	20–30	South America

Main vertebrate host	Whether pathogenic (+) or not (−) in man and domestic stock	Invertebrate host	
		Main vectors	Mechanical transmitters
cattle, sheep, deer and equines	+ in equines, cattle and sheep	Glossina morsitans and tachinoides	biting dipterans
cattle, sheep, deer and equines	+ in equines, cattle and sheep	—	biting dipterans
antelope, pigs, cattle sheep and goats	+ in pigs, sheep and cattle	various Glossina species	biting dipterans
antelope, sheep, cattle, pigs, dogs, equines and camels	+ in cattle, sheep, goats and equines (NAGANA)	Glossina morsitans austeni and longipalpalis	biting dipterans
warthogs, pigs and camels	+ in pigs	Glossina morsitans and brevipalpalis	biting dipterans
warthogs and pigs	+ in young pigs	Glossina brevipalpalis	unknown
antelope, equines, dogs, cattle, sheep, pigs and goats	+ in equines, sheep, dogs and goats	Glossina morsitans palpalis and tachinoides	biting dipterans
man	+ in man (SLEEPING SICKNESS)	Glossina palpalis and tachinoides	biting dipterans
man, deer and cattle	+ in man (SLEEPING SICKNESS)	Glossina morsitans swynnertoni and pallidipes	biting dipterans
equines, cattle, goats, sheep and capybara	+ in horses (MAL DE CADERAS)	—	biting dipterans
equines, camels, deer, cattle, dogs and sheep	+ in equines (SURRA)	—	biting dipterans
equines	+ in equines (DOURINE)	—	biting dipterans (rare) (by copulation)

[*continued*]

	Subgenus	Species of Trypanosoma	Approx. length (μ m)	Geographical distribution
Stercoraria (posterior station development)	Megatrypanum	T. theileri	60–100	ubiquitous
		T. melophagium	40–60	ubiquitous
	Herpetosoma	T. rangeli	25–35	South America
		T. lewisi	20–35	ubiquitous
	Schizotrypanum	T. cruzi	15–25	Central and South America

mammals are passed from one host to another by arthropods. In the case of trypanosomes affecting man and his domesticated animals all of the transmitters have been found to be insects. Such insects usually act as vectors, that is they are true intermediate hosts in which cyclical development of the flagellates occurs. However, the insects may be non-cyclical (mechanical) transmitters in which case the disseminator, usually a biting dipterous fly, must have its feeding interrupted and pass quickly to another animal to complete its meal. If this occurs then blood from the first animal present on the proboscis of the insect may be injected into the second when feeding recommences. Should the transferred blood contain trypanosomes then, of course, these can be introduced into the lesion. If transmission is to be successful it is important that the time between the two feeds does not exceed about fifteen minutes, for after this time the blood on the proboscis containing the trypanosomes will have dried and consequently the flagellates will have perished.

Some species of trypanosomes are transmitted by non-cyclical means exclusively. For example, biting flies including members of

Main vertebrate host	Whether pathogenic (+) or not (−) in man and domestic stock	Invertebrate host Main vectors	Mechanical transmitters
cattle and antelope	−	*Tabanus* and *Haematopota* species	biting dipterans
sheep	−	*Melophagus ovinus*	biting dipterans
cats, dogs, opossums, monkeys and man	− (but pathogenic to vector)	*Rhodnius* and *Triatoma* species	biting dipterans
rats	−	*Nosopsyllus fasciatus*	biting dipterans
rodents, monkeys, opossums, armadillos and man	+ in man (CHAGAS'S DISEASE)	*Panstrongylus*, *Triatoma* and *Rhodnius* species	biting dipterans

the genera *Tabanus* and *Stomoxys* disseminate *T. evansi evansi*, *T. equinum* and *T. vivax viennei*, there being no vector of these protozoans.

T. equinum, the causative agent of 'mal de caderas' of horses in South America, and *T. evansi evansi*, the aetiological agent of 'surra' in Asia, the Far East, North Africa, Mauritius and Central and South America, are both thought to have evolved from *T. brucei brucei* by the movement of hosts outside of the tsetse fly belt of Africa. Subsequently, these species have become adapted to mechanical transmission with loss of the cycle in the vector. Similarly, *T. vivax viennei* occurs outside of the tsetse fly belt in Central and South America, Mauritius and the West Indies, where it causes a disease in cattle, sheep, goats and horses.

However, it is more normal for *Trypanosoma* species to be passed from one host to another by both cyclical and non-cyclical means, with the latter being the more important and more usual.

T. vivax vivax, which has similar hosts and pathogenicity to *T. v. viennei* but which is found throughout East, West and Central Africa, may be transmitted mechanically, but is usually passed from

L

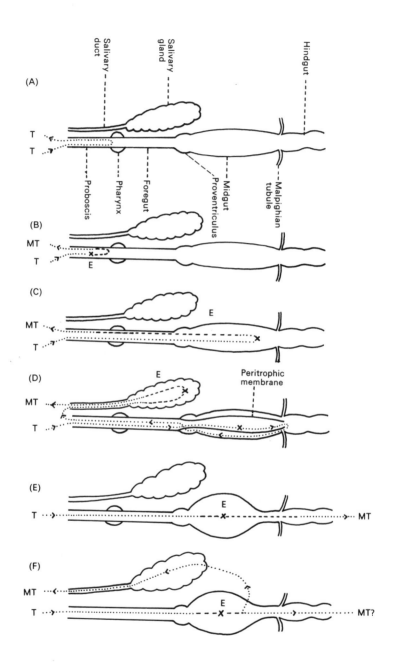

host to host following development in the tsetse flies, *Glossina morsitans* and *G. tachinoides*. In the fly the cycle occurs in the proboscis only (Fig. 118 B), with the ingested trypomastigote forms multiplying by longitudinal fission before becoming epimastigotes which later revert to trypomastigotes. These final stages are morphologically similar to the ingested trypomastigotes, but are described as 'metacyclic' as they have completed a cycle of development within the vector. When the infected tsetse fly bites some metacyclic trypomastigotes are regurgitated into the wound.

In the African species *T. congolense* and *T. simiae* a more complex development in the tsetse vector is shown. Here the imbibed trypomastigotes multiply in the midgut of the tsetse and later migrate forwards; in so doing they pass through the epimastigote stage before reverting to the metacyclic trypomastigote form (Fig. 118 C). The geographical distribution and major vectors of *T. congolense* and *T. simiae* are given in Table 8.

An even more complex cycle is shown in the tsetse vector in the case of *T. suis* and the *T. brucei* subspecies, viz. *T. brucei brucei*, *T. b. rhodesiense* and *T. b. gambiense*. In these flagellates the ingested trypomastigotes pass to the midgut where longitudinal division takes place. The newly divided forms eventually pass back into the hindgut region (see Fig. 119) where they remain for a short time only before entering the space between the gut wall and the peritrophic membrane (ectoperitrophic space). Within this cavity they move anteriorly until they reach the proventriculus

Figure 118 Life cycles of trypanosomes in their invertebrate transmitters:
A, mechanical on or in proboscis of biting flies, e.g. *Trypanosoma vivax viennei*;
B, development in proboscis of *Glossina* species, e.g. *T. vivax vivax*;
C, development in the midgut and proboscis of *Glossina* species, e.g. *T. congolense*;
D, development in the midgut and salivary glands of *Glossina* species, e.g. *T. brucei rhodesiense*;
E, development in the midgut and hindgut of *Rhodnius* species, e.g. *T. cruzi*;
F, development in the midgut and either salivary glands or hindgut of *Rhodnius* species, e.g. *T. rangeli*.
Key to diagram :   X denotes phase of multiplication,
                     T denotes trypomastigote stage,
                    MT denotes metacyclic trypomastigote stage,
                     E denotes epimastigote stage.

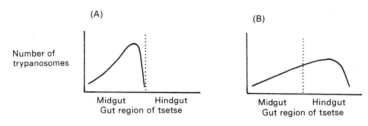

Figure 119 Distribution of trypanosomes A, before and B, after a blood meal. The peritrophic membrane terminates in the hindgut, and in order to enter the ectoperitrophic space the trypanosomes must enter the hindgut region. However, the hindgut pH is normally too acidic for the trypanosomes to enter, but changes to approximately that of the midgut after a meal when a dilute osmoregulatory fluid is passed into the hindgut from the Malpighian tubules. The purpose of osmoregulation is to remove excess water and salts from the body following the fluid meal.

where the membrane originates. In this region the membrane, which is newly formed, is soft and the trypomastigotes penetrate it to re-enter the lumen of the midgut (Fig. 120). Subsequently they migrate forward through the oesophagus, pharynx and proboscis to gain entry to the hypopharynx, which is an anterior extension of the common salivary duct. The flagellates continue their migrations via the salivary ducts to the salivary glands where they are now recognizable as epimastigotes. These attach to the walls of the glands by means of their flagella, divide by longitudinal fission, and then become metacyclic trypomastigotes which lie freely in the lumina of the salivary glands. When the tsetse fly feeds next the

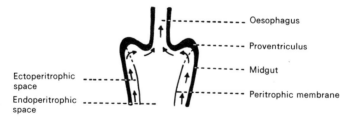

Figure 120 Proventricular region of a tsetse fly showing the migration route of trypanosomes, as shown by arrows. The soft, newly secreted peritrophic membrane is indicated by a dotted line.

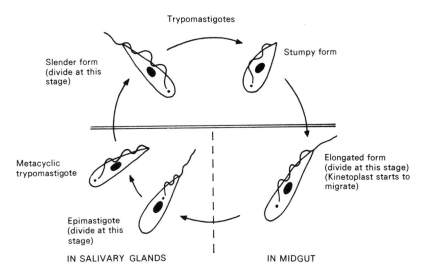

IN BLOOD OF MAMMAL

Trypomastigotes

Slender form
(divide at this
stage)

Stumpy form

Metacyclic
trypomastigote

Elongated form
(divide at this stage)
(Kinetoplast starts to
migrate)

Epimastigote
(divide at this
stage)

IN SALIVARY GLANDS

IN MIDGUT

Figure 121 Life cycle of the *Trypanosoma brucei* subspecies.

trypomastigotes are introduced into the host together with the salivary secretion.

The migration route of *T. brucei* subspecies is shown diagrammatically in Fig. 118 D and the morphological changes within the life cycle are depicted in Fig. 121. In particular, it should be noted that in the vertebrate blood-stream two morphological types of trypomastigote exist: the long, slender form with a distinct free flagellum and the short, stumpy form which lacks a free flagellum. Slender forms give rise to stumpy forms and a complete range of intermediates may be seen. It is the slender forms only which are capable of division in the blood.

Intensive studies have been made on *T. brucei* subspecies in order to explain the movement of the kinetoplast and associated locomotory organelles throughout the life cycle. These have revealed that the kinetoplast produces mitochondria with which it retains connection and that the kinetoplast contains deoxyribosenucleic acid (DNA). When the trypomastigote enters

the insect midgut the kinetoplast starts to produce a posterior
mitochondrion (Fig. 122) which thus pushes the kinetoplast, the
basal body and the flagellum anteriorly. This movement continues
until the kinetoplast and the associated locomotory organelles are
anterior to the nucleus, by which time the flagellate has arrived at
the salivary glands. This stage is referred to as the epimastigote
stage.

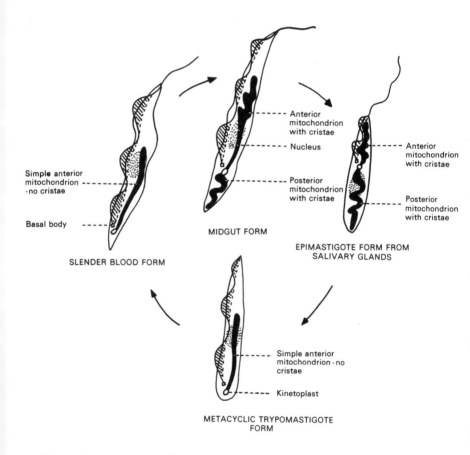

Figure 122 Changes occurring in the mitochondria of trypanosomes of the *brucei*
subgroup.

It is now recognized that the observed morphological changes are a reflection of physiological changes of the flagellate. Forms found in the midgut of the tsetse fly have been shown to respire aerobically utilizing Kreb's cycle and to perform hydrogen transfer by means of the cytochrome system. In contrast, the flagellates found in the blood of the mammalian host lack Kreb's cycle enzymes and cytochrome pigments. Instead their terminal respiration is by means of glycolysis, which occurs in small vesicles found throughout the cytoplasm of the protozoans. Glycolysis is a rather extravagant method of obtaining energy for each glucose molecule provides only two molecules of adenosine triphosphate (ATP), the end product of the reaction, pyruvic acid, still being rich in energy. However, such extravagance is permissable owing to the large amounts of available glucose in the surrounding medium. In contrast to this, in aerobic respiration the pyruvic acid is processed further to yield an additional thirty-six molecules of ATP, water and carbon dioxide remaining as end products of the reaction. This more economical method of glucose utilization is essential when the flagellate is in the tsetse's midgut, for in this site glucose is becoming scarce, particularly as digestion of the blood meal proceeds.

Mention has already been made of the conversion of slender to stumpy forms in the blood. Accompanying this change in shape is the activation of the mitochondrion when the Kreb's cycle enzymes are synthesized. Such forms are pre-adapted to survival in the tsetse's midgut and, in fact, are the only flagellates which are infective to the flies.

As noted above, in the salivary glands the epimastigotes, having completed their phase of multiplication, revert to trypomastigotes. These metacyclic forms resemble the stumpy flagellates in the blood of the vertebrate and are the only individuals which are infective to new vertebrate hosts. Why it should be that mitochondrial regression must occur for trypanosomes to become infective is at present unknown. When introduced into a vertebrate the metacyclic trypomastigotes become elongated (slender forms) which continue to lack enzymes for aerobic respiration.

Trypanosomes of the *T. brucei* subgroup cause serious diseases in man and his domesticated stock; these are discussed later in the chapter.

T. evansi equiperdum is thought to have evolved from *T. brucei brucei* by the movement of the host species (horses) outside of the tsetse fly belt. Instead of a mechanical transmitter filling the role of the disseminator this is brought about by contact of one horse with another during copulation. In this species the loss of a vector is accompanied by loss of the kinetoplast and *T. evansi equiperdum* is, in fact, unable to cycle owing to the inability to synthesize Kreb's cycle enzymes necessary for respiration in the insect vector. Although transmission by means of a biting dipteran is still possible it occurs only occasionally. *T. e. equiperdum* is found in both the blood and in oedematous patches on the skin of horses. Some patches occur on the genital organs and during copulation they may burst and liberate infective trypanosomes. These enter the body of the mating partner by way of a lesion of the skin, itself a common result of coitus.

A quite distinct variety of life history is found in trypanosomes of the section Stercoraria, for example *T. cruzi*, a parasite of man and other animals in Central and South America. In this species, as in other members of the section, the vector is an insect other than a tsetse fly. In the insect vector (*Rhodnius prolixus* and other reduviid bugs in the case of *T. cruzi*) trypomastigote stages taken up during feeding become epimastigotes which subsequently divide by longitudinal fission in the midgut, the newly formed flagellates passing backward to the hindgut to become infective metacyclic trypomastigotes (Fig. 118 E). Infection occurs when these are passed out of the bug together with the faeces. This takes place almost immediately after the completion of feeding and so trypanosomes are deposited close to the lesion caused by the bite of the insect. Quite often the insects bite around the eyes and so the infective faeces are easily rubbed into the eyes and may gain entry to the body through the intact conjunctiva. Alternatively, the trypanosomes may enter the body by way of the lesion of the bite or by the faeces being transferred to the conjunctiva by the person scratching the wound and then rubbing the eyes. Transmission of disease involving the faeces entering the body or being deposited on the body is referred to as contaminative transmission.

Following their injection into the vertebrate the trypomastigotes enter histiocytes in the skin and become amastigotes (Fig. 123). These multiply rapidly and the host reacts by producing a local inflammation. Subsequently they pass via the blood and lymphatic system to muscular tissues, often those of the heart and alimentary canal, where further multiplication occurs in the amastigote stage. These revert to trypomastigotes via promastigotes and epimastigotes which then escape from the host cell and circulate in the blood-stream. Eventually they re-enter muscle cells and become amastigote forms which divide once again.

In the closely related *T. theileri*, *T. lewisi* and *T. melophagium*,

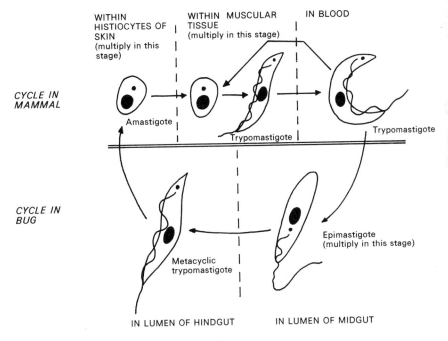

Figure 123 Life cycle of *Trypanosoma cruzi*.

which are non-pathogenic trypanosomes of cattle, rats and sheep respectively, the cycle in the vector is basically similar to that described for *T. cruzi*. However, the metacylic trypomastigotes are introduced by the flies *Tabanus* and *Haematopota* in the former case; the rat fleas *Nosopsyllus fasciatus* and *Xenopsylla cheopis* in the case of *T. lewisi*; and the ked *Melophagus ovinus* in the example of the flagellate *T. melophagium*. In the vertebrate host the cycle occurs in the blood only, with the introduced trypomastigotes undergoing morphological change and dividing as epimastigotes.

T. rangeli shows a variation on the above theme. This flagellate, which occurs non-pathogenically in man and other animals in South America, is taken up by the vector (*Rhodnius* and *Triatoma* species) as a trypomastigote stage and passes to the midgut where it becomes an epimastigote. Multiplication follows and after reverting to trypomastigotes the flagellates either pass backward to the midgut (contended by some authorities) or migrate through the midgut wall, traverse the haemocoel and enter the salivary glands (Fig. 118 F).

Infections of man and domesticated animals
Sleeping sickness (African trypanosomiasis)   This is a disease of man caused by subspecies of *T. brucei*. Two diseases are recognized, viz. Gambian and Rhodesian sleeping sickness, which are similar with regard to the course of infection and symptoms although in the latter the causative agent is more virulent and the progress of the disease more rapid. If untreated both diseases are fatal.

The aetiological agent of Gambian sleeping sickness, which occurs in West and Central Africa, is *T. brucei gambiense*, while the Rhodesian disease of East and Central Africa is caused by *T. brucei rhodesiense*. In the initial stages of infection when the trypanosomes are circulating the symptoms include fever and headaches, accompanied by weakness, lethargy and lymph gland enlargement. The symptoms may clear up at this stage, although persistent trypanosomes may enter the cerebro-spinal fluid by way of adjacent blood vessels. At this stage the characteristic symptoms of 'sleeping sickness' are seen, i.e. sleepiness turns to stupor and ends in a coma and death. Untreated cases of *T. b. gambiense* may last for several years before death ensues, but *T. b. rhodesiense* infections proceed rapidly and the circulating stages are extremely toxic and may kill the host before the central nervous system becomes involved.

Prior to the involvement of the nervous system the chance of recovery following administration of the drug *suramin* is good. However, following the invasion of the cerebro-spinal fluid prognosis is less certain; in this set of circumstances *suramin* is used in combination with an arsenical such as *tryparsamide* and *melarsoprol*.

Chagas's disease (American trypanosomiasis)   Once *T. cruzi* has been introduced into the human host, usually via the eyes, there follows a phase of multiplication which is accompanied by a host reaction comprising local swelling and the enlargement of adjacent lymph glands. As the trypanosomes usually enter through the eye it is often the eyelids, conjunctiva and one side of the face which swell and the glands on that side of the neck which become enlarged. The toxic by-products of metabolism of these tissue forms are circulated in the blood-stream, producing headaches and fever.

As the disease progresses muscular tissues become invaded, and this may lead to their being weakened or even destroyed. The heart is frequently the muscle attacked and thus heart disorders are a common symptom of this disease. Other symptoms which develop are general lymph gland, spleen and liver hypertrophy and anaemia. There is no known cure for this disease which may eventually be fatal.

Dourine (equine trypanosomiasis)   Following transferences of *T. evansi equiperdum* to a horse during coitus the first symptoms are those of urethral or vaginal discharge of mucus, oedema of the genitalia and fever. The oedema spreads over much of the ventral

surface, which is followed by the appearance of deeper
oedematous patches under the skin surface, not necessarily
confined to the venter of the animal. Paralysis follows and the
disease may terminate in death.

Surra (equine trypanosomiasis)   The most obvious symptoms of
this disease are emaciation and oedema of various parts of the body
surface. There may be intermittent fever, anaemia and enlargement
of the lymph glands and spleen. Once again, death often results
from this disease, the causative agent of which is *T. evansi evansi.*

Mal de Caderas (equine trypanosomiasis)   This is caused by
T. equinum and is manifested by emaciation, followed by weakness
of the hind limbs. This weakness spreads to the remainder of the
animal leading to total loss of locomotory ability. Oedematous
patches appear on the anterior regions of the body, and anaemia
and spleen and lymph node enlargement follow. Again, the disease
is often fatal.

Nagana (bovine trypanosomiasis)   The disease produced by
T. congolense may be acute, in which case death occurs within
two to three months, or chronic, with full recovery after about a
year. Both forms of the disease produce swellings of the lymph
nodes, anaemia and emaciation. In the acute disease haemorrhages
occur in the heart muscle and the bone marrow becomes depleted.
     Many people also refer to the disease caused by *T. brucei brucei*
as nagana. This disease is most acute in horses but also attacks
dogs, goats, sheep, pigs and cattle. In the majority of infections
pigs and cattle show few symptoms but the remaining hosts
succumb with symptoms of fever, lethargy, anaemia, muscular
weakness and oedema of the skin of the limbs and abdomen. The
disease is invariably fatal.

11

Other diseases caused by insect-borne Protozoa and microorganisms

In this chapter the better-known insect-transmitted protozoans, bacteria, rickettsiae, viruses and spirochaetes, apart from those transmitted by mosquitoes and sandflies, will receive attention. These include many diseases which are carried almost exclusively by insects, for example the infamous plague, and others like poliomyelitis and amoebiasis for which arthropods act as mechanical transmitters to provide an additional method of propagation.

Protozoan parasites

In earlier chapters mention is made of *Leishmania*, *Trypanosoma* and *Plasmodium*, three particularly important genera of protozoan parasites. In this section three close relatives of the malarial parasites will be discussed, all of which have insects as their intermediate hosts; they are *Haemoproteus* and *Leucocytozoon*, both parasitic in birds, and *Hepatocystis*, a parasite of mammals. Additionally, insects may transport the cysts of certain protozoans, like *Entamoeba histolytica* and *Giardia lamblia*, from human excreta to the food of a new human host. Such cysts may be carried adhering to the body surface of such flies as *Musca domestica* or they may pass unharmed through the alimentary canal or be regurgitated by coprophagous insects following their ingestion from faeces.

Haemoproteus columbae is a parasite of domestic and wild pigeons and some other species of wild birds throughout the world. The life cycle of this parasite is similar to that of *Plasmodium*, with several modifications (Fig. 124). Gametocytes are found in red

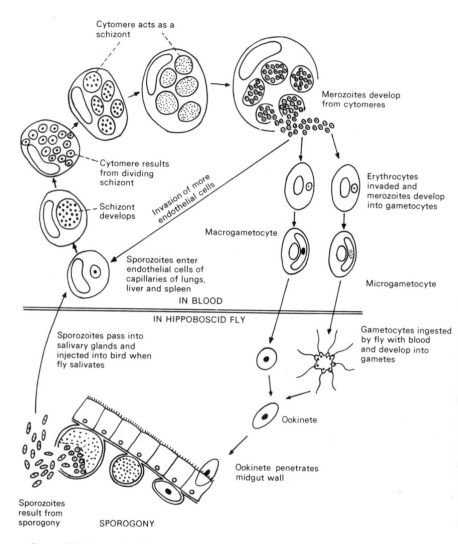

Cytomere acts as a schizont

Cytomere results from dividing schizont

Invasion of more endothelial cells

Schizont develops

Merozoites develop from cytomeres

Erythrocytes invaded and merozoites develop into gametocytes

Macrogametocyte

Microgametocyte

Sporozoites enter endothelial cells of capillaries of lungs, liver and spleen

IN BLOOD

IN HIPPOBOSCID FLY

Sporozoites pass into salivary glands and injected into bird when fly salivates

Gametocytes ingested by fly with blood and develop into gametes

Ookinete

Ookinete penetrates midgut wall

Sporozoites result from sporogony

SPOROGONY

Figure 124 Life cycle of *Haemoproteus columbae.*

blood cells of the host and are ingested by the hippoboscid flies
Pseudolynchia canariensis, Ornithomyia avicularia and others. It is
possible that a species of *Culicoides* is also involved in the

transmission of this *Haemoproteus* species. In the fly exflagellation occurs and following fertilization the ookinete penetrates the midgut wall and, as in *Plasmodium*, lies between the cell layer and the basement membrane. Here sporogony takes place and the resultant sporozoites pass to the salivary glands and are transferred to a new host when the fly bites. In the bird the sporozoites penetrate endothelial cells lining blood capillaries of the lungs, liver, spleen and other organs and develop into schizonts. However, each schizont breaks up into about fifteen small, uninucleate bodies called cytomeres. Each cytomere then acts as a schizont itself and produces numerous merozoites which either re-invade endothelial cells to undergo repeated schizogony cycles or penetrate erythrocytes to develop into gametocytes. *Haemoproteus columbae* does not produce a disease in adult birds but young birds may die of anaemia and interstitial pneumonia with enlargement of the liver and spleen.

Other haemoproteids worthy of mention here are *Haemoproteus lophortyx*, a common parasite of quail in North America transmitted by the hippoboscids *Lynchia hirsuta* and *Stilbometopa impressa*, and *Haemoproteus nettionis* (placed by some authorities in the genus *Parahaemoproteus*), of domestic and wild ducks, geese and swans in most parts of the world. The vector of this latter parasite is a *Culicoides* species, most likely *C. piliferus*, although the exact identification of the vector species has not as yet been made.

The genus *Leucocytozoon* also has affinities with the malarial parasites and hence, not surprisingly, shares many common features with regard to its life cycle. In *L. simondi* of geese and ducks in Europe, North America and Asia the cycle in the vectors *Simulium rugglesi* and *S. parnassum* follow the pattern of *Plasmodium* in *Anopheles*, except that the oocyst develops within an epithelial cell of the midgut and that the salivary glands are invaded by only a few sporozoites, the remainder presumably entering the proboscis directly. On being introduced into the bird by a bite of an infected fly the sporozoites enter a cycle of schizogony in the lymphoid-macrophage cells of the spleen, liver

and heart. The merozoites which result from schizogony take one of
three courses: some enter erythrocytes and mature to gametocytes,
while others invade either liver parenchyma cells to produce
cytomeres which eventually give rise to more merozoites or
lymphoid-macrophage cells in the spleen, lungs, heart, liver and
other organs to form very large schizonts called megaloschizonts.
The latter develop into cytomeres and then merozoites, which
finally invade blood cells (probably lymphocytes) to develop into
gametocytes. However, the host blood cell is so distorted that it is
difficult to determine whether it is a red or a white cell which is
being parasitized (Fig. 125). *Leucocytozoon simondi* is pathogenic
to young birds, causing high mortality due in the main to the
presence of megaloschizonts in vital organs and blood cell
destruction.

Leucocytozoon smithi of turkeys in Europe and North America
and *L. sakharoffi* of birds of the crow family in Europe, America,
India and Australia exhibit a similar life cycle to that of *L. simondi*.
However, in the former species *Simulium occidentale* and other
species of the genus have been incriminated as vectors, while
L. sakharoffi has been found to be cycled by *Simulium aureum* and
S. latipes.

A number of species of the mammalian parasite *Hepatocystis*
exist, the best documented of which is *H. kochi* of African
monkeys. The life histories of members of this genus are
reminiscent of *Plasmodium* but, once again, several modifications
occur. To begin with the vectors are not mosquitoes but are midges
of the genus *Culicoides*, for example *C. adersi*, and following
fertilization of the macrogamete by the microgamete in the midgut

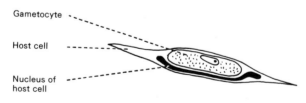

Figure 125 Gametocyte of *Leucocytozoon simondi*.

of the fly the ookinete passes right through the midgut wall and is transported in the haemolymph to the head of the midge. In this location the ookinete secretes a thin cyst wall and is then known as an oocyst, which undergoes a cycle of sporogony, the end product of which are sporozoites. Following their release into the haemocoel the sporozoites invade the proboscis apparently directly and not by way of the salivary glands, a phenomenon which seems to occur also in *Leucocytozoon*.

Bacteria

In the main the role of insects in the dissemination of bacterial diseases is one of passive carriage. When feeding on excreta coprophagous insects either ingest bacilli or the bacilli become attached to their bodies. If the flies then alight on foodstuffs the bacteria may be transferred by contact, regurgitated or deposited together with the fly's faeces. Although in some instances multiplication of the bacteria occurs in the insect vector, as in plague, true cyclical development in the invertebrate host is lacking among the insect-borne bacteria.

Table 9 shows those bacterial diseases for which insects have been shown to aid in transmission. In most of these, however, dissemination can be effected without the assistance of an insect, although some, like plague, normally require a vector for their propagation.

Plague has a long history of epidemics, for example during the fourteenth and seventeenth centuries in Europe. Now plague has natural foci in many widespread places, among them being Asia, the Far East, East and Central Africa, South America and western USA. In all of these locations plague is a zoonosis and is enzootic in wild rodents. Both the brown rat, *Rattus rattus norvegicus*, and the black rat, *R. rattus rattus*, are instrumental in passing the disease to man, the latter rodent being a close companion of man in towns and cities. When inoculated into the skin of man by a flea the aetiological agent, *Pasteurella pestis*, passes in lymph channels to lymph nodes and produces inflammation and enlargement of the

Table 9 The principal insect-borne bacterial diseases of man and domesticated animals

Disease and host if other than man	Causative agent	Vectors and notes
Anthrax (cattle, equines, sheep, goats and man)	*Bacillus anthracis*	Various coprophagous insects spread spores (e.g. *Musca domestica*) and haematophagous insects transmit it mechanically (e.g. *Tabanus* and *Stomoxys*).
Botulism	*Clostridium botulinum*	Transmitted mechanically by larvae and adults of *Piophila casei* (cheese fly).
Cholera	*Vibrio comma* (=*V. cholerae*)	House flies (e.g. *Musca domestica*) and cockroaches may contaminate human food after feeding on faeces from infected persons.
Dysenteries Note: dysentery may also be caused by protozoans (for example *Entamoeba histolytica* and *Balantidium coli*) and by helminths (*Schistosoma* and *Oesophagostomum* species).	*Shigella* species, for example *S. dysenteriae* and *S. sonnei*	Many flies, cockroaches, even wasps which have fed on infected flies, can transport dysentery bacilli from faeces to food. The main flies involved are *Calliphora erythrocephala*, *Fannia scalaris*, *F. canicularis* and *Musca domestica*.
Gastro-enteritis	*Escherichia coli*	Various flies (e.g. *Lucilia sericata*, *Musca domestica* and *Fannia canicularis*) carry bacilli from faeces to food.

Disease and host if other than man	Causative agent	Vectors and notes
Enteric fevers	*Salmonella typhi* (typhoid); *S. paratyphi* and *S. schottmulleri* (paratyphoid fevers); *S. enteritidis* (food poisoning)	Carried by house flies, cockroaches and other insects from either faeces or urine of an infected person to human food.
Plague (see text)	*Pasteurella pestis*	Fleas, notably *Xenopsylla cheopis* and *Nosopsyllus fasciatus*
Tularaemia	*Brucella* (= *Pasteurella*) *tularensis*	A zoonosis maintained by birds, rodents and lagomorphs, it is primarily a tick-borne disease, but many blood-sucking insects transmit it mechanically and by contamination.
Other brucelloses (goats and sheep; cattle respectively)	*Brucella melitensis* and *B. abortus*	Various blood-sucking insects transmit the bacilli when feeding. Both parasites can be transferred to man in milk from goats and cows. *B. abortus* is the cause of parasitic abortion in cows.
Bovine mastitis (cattle)	*Streptococcus agalactiae*	Transmitted by regurgitation and in the excreta of flies, notably *Musca domestica*, the bacillus is picked up from infected udders and passed to the same site in uninfected cows.

lymph glands, a condition known as bubonic plague. This may
then be followed by bacterial invasion of the blood-stream
(septicemic plague) and other organs, in particular the lungs
(pneumonic plague).

Pneumonic plague may also be contracted directly from an
infected person by respiratory contamination, whereby bacteria pass
from person to person in breath and respiratory droplets. As a
consequence of this method of infection lobular pneumonia, similar
to influenza pneumonia, occurs, usually with fatal results. The
epidemiological picture for plague transmission to man may
therefore be expressed as indicated in Fig. 126.

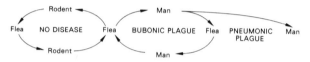

Figure 126 Transmission pattern of plague.

In severe cases of plague the mucous membranes and skin
develop dark red patches as a result of local haemorrhage; this
explains the common name for the disease of 'black death'.
Except in treated cases the mortality rate in plague infections is
very high. The treatment involves the administration of certain
drugs, for example *streptomycin* and *sulphamerazine*. Vaccines
prepared from either killed, virulent forms of the bacillus or living,

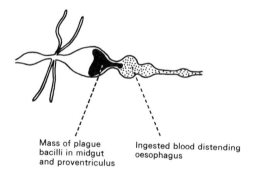

Mass of plague
bacilli in midgut
and proventriculus

Ingested blood distending
oesophagus

Figure 127 Gut of flea showing blockage caused by a mass of plague bacilli.

avirulent strains give protection, not by preventing the disease from being acquired but by minimizing the symptoms following infection.

The gut of a flea showing the blockage caused by multiplication of bacilli is depicted in Fig. 127, and a number of bacilli in the blood of a human are shown in Fig. 128.

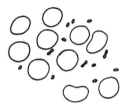

Figure 128 Plague bacilli in a blood smear.

Rickettsiae

It is usual to recognize five distinct groups of rickettsial organisms, two of which concern us here in that they are insect-borne. The remaining three groupings, namely the spotted fever group, the tsutsugamushi group and the Q-fever group are all transmitted by acarines (ticks and mites).

Typhus group of rickettsiae

To this group belong two important organisms which cause louse-borne typhus fever and murine typhus in man. The former disease results from the presence of *Rickettsia prowazekii*, which is transmitted by the human lice *Pediculus humanus corporis* and, occasionally, *P. humanus humanus* in nearly all parts of the world. The louse picks up the rickettsiae when feeding on infected humans and the organisms invade the insect's midgut cells where they multiply. Eventually the parasitized cells burst to liberate the rickettsiae into the gut lumen, and these are subsequently excreted. If the insect's faeces together with their contained rickettsiae are rubbed into a skin lesion, or even if the whole insect is crushed on to broken skin, then the organisms gain entry to the human body

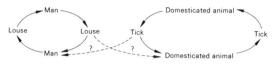

Figure 129 Transmission pattern of louse-borne typhus fever.

and an infection commences. The rickettsiae are highly pathogenic to man and cause high mortality. Having entered the skin they invade endothelial cells of capillaries throughout the body, particularly in the skin, and give rise to an extensive rash. Later symptoms include chills and fevers, delirium and broncho-pneumonia. Cure of this disease is effected by the administration of *chloramphenicol* and certain other related drugs.

It is of interest that this rickettsia also causes the death of the louse host some twelve or so days after their initial infection, a point which contrasts with murine typhus (see below) which has no ill effect on the flea host.

Louse-borne typhus is probably a zoonosis with domesticated animals acting as reservoir hosts. The epidemiological picture for this disease is complicated by the fact that other arthropods, for example the tick *Amblyomma variegatum*, can transmit the disease to domesticated animals although whether the tick is responsible for infecting man and the louse for infecting domesticated animals is not certain. The transmission of the rickettsia can be expressed as shown in Fig. 129.

Murine (flea-borne) typhus is a disease related to louse-borne typhus, the aetiological agent being *Rickettsia prowazekii* var. *mooseri*, otherwise known as either *Rickettsia mooseri* or *R. typhi*. Murine typhus has a worldwide distribution, but is particularly common in North America, and produces a mild disease of mice and rats. Occasionally it is passed to man, giving rise to an illness similar to louse-borne typhus although far less severe. With regard to vectors of *R. prowazekii* var. *mooseri*, it has been shown that the fleas *Xenopsylla cheopis*, *X. astia* and *Nosopsyllus fasciatus* and the rat louse *Polyplax spinulosus* transfer the parasite from rodent to rodent and that the fleas may pass the rickettsiae to man as indicated in Fig. 130.

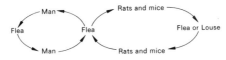

Figure 130 Transmission pattern of flea-borne typhus fever.

Trench fever group of rickettsiae
The organism responsible for producing the type disease (i.e.
trench fever) is *Rickettsia quintana,* transmitted in parts of Europe,
Mexico, Algeria, Ethiopia and China by the body louse
Pediculus humanus corporis. Lice pick up the organisms when they
feed on infected humans and the rickettsiae adhere to the cuticular
margin of the midgut epithelium where they multiply. The site of
multiplication is thus different from that of *R. prowazekii* as it is
extracellular and not within gut cells as in the louse-borne typhus
rickettsiae.

Following the contamination of skin wounds with louse faeces
man shows symptoms of aches and pains with intermittent fever.
The disease incapacitates but is not fatal and can be treated by the
drug *chloramphenicol,* also used in the treatment of the typhus
fevers.

Arboviruses
The arthropod-borne viruses multiply in both susceptable vertebrate
and invertebrate hosts and are transferred from one to the other
when insects ingest infected blood and subsequently salivate.

Arboviruses are divided into three major groups, as mentioned in
chapter 8. As far as is known all members of group A are
mosquito-borne while those of group B are either mosquito- or
tick-borne. Acarine-borne diseases are beyond the scope of the
present text and are not discussed here, but the insect-borne A and
B group viruses are listed in chapter 8, where yellow fever and
dengue from group B are given fuller treatment. Viruses of group C
are transmitted by various vectors: mosquitoes, tabanid flies,
sandflies, ticks and mites. The sandfly-transmitted papatacii fever
and the mosquito-disseminated diseases have already been noted;

here two more important viruses will be commented upon, namely
vesicular stomatitis virus of equines, bovines and man in Central
America and parts of North and South America, the mechanical
transmitters of which are various tabanid flies and mosquitoes (e.g.
Tabanus trispilus and *Culex tarsalis*), and human poliomyelitis virus
which is carried by non-haematophagous flies (e.g. *Musca
domestica* and *Phormia regina*). The flies pick up the latter virus
from faeces of infected persons, sewage and corpses of victims of
the disease and carry them on their body surfaces, particularly their
legs, where the virus not only persists for several weeks but
apparently multiplies. When such a fly alights on food or on sores
and wounds on the body human infections follow.

Spirochaetes

The most important of the insect-transmitted spirochaetes is
Borrelia recurrentis which is found in the body fluids of man in
parts of the Middle East. It does not invade cells but causes tissue
damage indirectly by the production of toxic metabolic by-
products. Symptoms of the disease commence with chills and
fevers which are followed by aches and pains, accompanied by
haemorrhage into the skin, anaemia and jaundice due to the
destruction of erythrocytes and liver cells. Recurrent fevers occur in
untreated cases but the administration of *streptomycin* or *penicillin*
alleviates the symptoms.

   B. recurrentis is transmitted by the louse *Pediculus humanus
corporis*. The spirochaetes are taken up from the blood of an
infected person (Fig. 131) by the louse and pass through its midgut

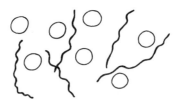

Figure 131 Spirochaetes in a blood smear.

wall into the haemocoel, from which site they become distributed throughout the body of the insect and subsequently multiply in its tissues. The spirochaetes never return to the alimentary canal of the louse and thus cannot be transferred by the bite of the insect but only by an infected insect being crushed on to the broken skin of a susceptible host. Transmission is thus not due to a natural activity of the louse but is initiated by accidental or human means.

Treponema pertenue, the aetiological agent of yaws, has already been noted in connection with mosquitoes, and here it is only necessary to add that it can also be transmitted mechanically by certain muscid flies.

12

Other insect-borne helminth diseases

'Helminth' is a collective name given to the Platyhelminthes, the Nematoda and the Acanthocephala, the separate characteristics of which are given on pages 195–6. In the section dealing with mosquito-borne diseases *Wuchereria bancrofti, Brugia malayi* and *Dirofilaria immitis* and *Setaria equina* are discussed and in the present chapter some other helminths of major importance are mentioned.

The role of insects in the dissemination of helminth parasites is, in fact, twofold. First, they may be mechanical transmitters, carrying eggs of parasites from the excreta in which they are voided to the food of their definitive host, and, second, they may act as true intermediate hosts in which cyclical development of the parasites takes place.

In the first of the above categories may be included a large number of nematodes, cestodes and digenoids whose eggs are transported by domestic dipterans such as *Musca domestica*. The more important of these parasites are listed in Table 10.

As well as acting as passive distributors, insects play a vital role in the life cycles of many parasites as intermediate hosts. Numerous examples of such relationships exist, but here only the better-known examples will be quoted, with several of these being discussed in detail.

Nematoda

A number of fairly distinct types of life cycle can be identified among members of the insect-borne Nematoda. In the filarial worms (order Filaroidea) a typical life cycle involves the production of microfilarial larvae which are ingested by an ectoparasitic insect

Table 10 Some helminth parasites mechanically transmitted by insects

Taxonomic group	Species	Main hosts	Geographical distribution
Nematoda	*Ancylostoma duodenale*	man	South Europe, North Africa and Asia
	Ascaris lumbricoides	man	worldwide
	Enterobius vermicularis	man	worldwide, but rare in tropics
	Necator americanus	man	America, Africa and South Asia
	Trichuris trichiura	man	worldwide
Cestoda	*Echinococcus granulosus*	man and dog	most parts of the world
	Taenia saginata	man and cattle	worldwide

and which develop in the tissues of the arthropod, moulting twice, to form infective third-stage larvae. These larvae pass forward to the mouthparts of the insect, from which site they are liberated when the arthropod next feeds.

In contrast to this, members of most other nematode orders rely on the intermediate host ingesting eggs (or occasionally larvae) passed out in the faeces or other body exudates of the host. In such intermediate hosts the eggs hatch in the gut and the emergent larvae pass through the gut wall into the haemocoel, where they invariably become encapsulated owing to a host reaction. Within the capsule the larva develops into the infective stage and awaits transference to the final host. In most cases the life cycle is

completed when the definitive host swallows the infected insect
and the worms escape from their capsules to infect their new host.
However, in, for example, *Habronema* and *Thelazia* (see later) the
infective larvae are not encapsulated but migrate to the insect's
proboscis and escape on to the host as the insect feeds.

Nematodes parasitic in man

Loa loa   This is the notorious 'eye worm' of man in the Congo,
Nigeria and the Cameroons which has been shown to be
transmitted during the feeding period of several tabanid flies of the
genus *Chrysops*, notably *C. silacea* and *C. dimidiata*. When such
flies feed they take up microfilariae of *Loa loa* with their blood meal
and on reaching the mesenteron of the insect the worms lose their
sheaths and quickly penetrate the midgut wall. Once inside the
haemocoel they enter a cell in the fat body and grow rapidly to
such an extent that within about two days they have outgrown the
cell and after ten days the worms have moulted twice to become
infective third-stage larvae which migrate through the haemocoel to
the head region.

The migratory route from the abdomen to the thorax is by way of
the narrow haemocoelic space at the junction of the thorax and
abdomen, and movement from the thorax to the head is via the
restricted haemolymph channels located between the tracheal
trunks and various other body organs. Once in the head region they
pass forward into the subcibarial haemocoel which lies just above
the insect's proboscis.

When the fly next feeds the infective larvae emerge from the
labio-hypopharyngeal membrane, a situation which contrasts
directly with that in *Wuchereria bancrofti* and *Brugia malayi*
escaping from mosquitoes and *Onchocerca volvulus* leaving
Simulium, where the point of exit is the tip of the labium (see page
122). The labio-hypopharyngeal membrane connects the base of the
labium with the base of the hypopharynx and becomes taut when
the fly feeds (Fig. 132), such tension on the membrane causing its
rupture in infected flies and hence the release of the nematode
larvae. The reason for the rupture is not completely clear, but it is

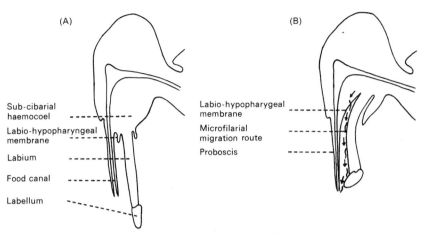

Figure 132 Longitudinal sections through the head of Chrysops to show the position of the labium and labio-hypopharyngeal membrane and the migratory route of microfilariae in A, a non-feeding fly and B, a feeding fly.

suggested that on feeding the gut distends and this causes the pressure to rise in the adjacent haemolymph. This pressure change is transferred to the head and breaks the membrane on attaining a critical value. Such a lesion does not appear to occur in uninfected flies and it is envisaged that it is the bulk of the nematode larvae in the haemocoel which is responsible for the pressure rising above the critical level.

Following their release on to the skin of the definitive host the worms burrow and subsequently migrate through subdermal connective tissues, including the anterior chamber of the eye. Normally these migrations cause no harm but may produce transient oedemas, called Calabar swellings, in any part of the body. The worms mature within about a year in subcutaneous tissues and female worms release microfilarial larvae which migrate between the subdermal tissues and the peripheral blood with a periodicity which coincides with the diurnal biting activity of the tabanid flies (Fig. 133).

The treatment of loiasis may take the form of either surgical removal of the worms or the administration of chemotherapeutics, for example diethylcarbamazine.

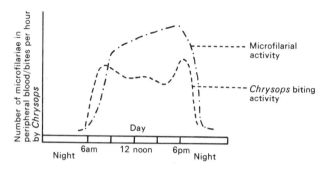

Figure 133 The biting activity of *Chrysops* and the periodicity of microfilariae of *Loa loa*.

Onchocerca volvulus   Onchocerciasis or 'river blindness' is the debilitating disease caused by this filarial worm throughout most parts of tropical Africa and the Yemen, and in parts of Central and South America. *O. volvulus* is a parasite of spider monkeys and gorillas as well as man, and the disease which it causes is therefore, strictly speaking, termed a zoonosis although man is by far the most common host. It has been suggested that the American and the African forms of this worm are distinct races or strains, and indeed it is likely that there may be a considerable number of varieties of this nematode within each of these continents.

Adult worms are found within characteristic nodules of subcutaneous connective tissue and the sheathless, non-periodic microfilariae are released into the fluid of this nodule and into the surrounding skin. *Simulium* species have been implicated as vectors of onchocerciasis, the major vector throughout Africa being *S. damnosum*, aided by members of the *S. neavei* complex in East Africa and *S. woodi* in Tanzania. In Central and South America *S. callidum*, *S. metallicum* and *S. ochraceum* have been shown to act as vectors of this disease. *Simulium* species are day-biters and possess a short proboscis which is well adapted for abstracting microfilariae from the skin for it penetrates just deep enough to remove larvae from below the epidermis. This, of course, implies that *Simulium* feeds on skin tissue fluids as well as on blood.

When a *Simulium* fly feeds on an infected host it ingests

microfilariae; these penetrate the peritrophic membrane lining the midgut and then the wall of the gut itself. The microfilariae are thus in the insect's haemocoel and travel to the thoracic musculature where they moult twice to become infective third-stage larvae which leave the muscle to migrate to the labium. After being released on to the skin surface the microfilariae penetrate to reach the subcutaneous tissues where they mature. As far as clinical symptoms are concerned, it is of note that it is the larvae and not the adults which are causative agents, a fact which contrasts with the situation in *Wuchereria* and *Brugia* where the adults cause the damage. The symptoms of onchocerciasis start with itching and a rash which is followed by thickening and later atrophy of the skin with loss of elasticity, a condition which may occasionally cause 'hanging groin' and hernias. Apart from skin diseases *Onchocerca volvulus* may on rare occasions produce elephantiasis due to the blockage of lymphatic vessels and blindness due to the formation of lesions and subsequent tissue reactions in the eye.

Treatment of onchocerciasis involves surgical removal of nodules and the administration of certain drugs, for example *suramin*, which kills both adult worms and microfilariae.

In addition to *O. volvulus* there are various species of *Onchocerca* in cattle and horses in all parts of the world which apparently cause no ill effects on their hosts. Examples of these are *O. gutturosa* in cattle in England transmitted by *Simulium ornatum* and *O. cervicalis* in European horses which is disseminated by the midge *Culicoides nubeculosus*.

Mansonella ozzardi   This parasite has a similar life cycle to *Onchocerca* and occurs, usually embedded in adipose tissues, in the body cavities of man in South America and the West Indies. The vectors of this parasite are the midges *Culicoides furens* and *C. paraenis*. *Mansonella ozzardi* causes few symptoms in man and little tissue reaction.

Dipetalonema (=Acanthocheilonema) perstans   Both man and apes may be infected with this worm, which develops in the peritoneum and which, although rarely pathogenic, can produce liver disorders. Details of the life cycle of this species are similar to those for other filarial worms, the implicated vectors being *Culicoides austeni* and *C. grahami*. *Dipetalonema perstans* is distributed throughout Central Africa, Guyana and New Guinea.

Nematodes of non-human hosts

Hartertia gallinarum   Fowl and bustards in many parts of Africa are the definitive hosts of this intestinal parasite. The intermediate hosts are worker termites, often of the genus *Macrohodothermes*, which ingest eggs from the faeces of the bird host. Immature stages of the parasite develop in the body cavity of the termite, and birds gain the disease by eating the infected insects.

Subulura brumpti   This is a parasite of the caecum of turkeys, fowl and other wild birds in parts of Europe, Africa and South America. The intermediate host of this avian parasite is either a beetle, for example *Dermestes* species, or a cockroach like *Blatella germanica*, which must be ingested by the bird for transmission to take place.

Spirocerca lupi   Eggs of this worm are voided from the definitive host in the excreta and must be ingested by coprophagous beetles, for example *Scarabeus* species, for the life cycle to continue. When the definitive hosts ingest such beetles they become infected. *Spirocerca lupi* is a parasite of dogs, foxes and wolves in many tropical and subtropical lands, being located in the oesophagus and the stomach wall.

Gongylonema pulchrum   *G. pulchrum* is distributed throughout most parts of the world and occurs in the oesophagus and rumen wall of sheep, cattle and other ungulates, and has been reported from man. The life cycle is typical of non-filarial worms and the intermediate host, a coprophagous beetle (e.g. *Blaps* species), must be ingested by the final host for the life cycle to continue.

Acuaria hamulosa   Infections of this parasite are found in the gizzard of turkeys and fowl in most countries, the birds becoming

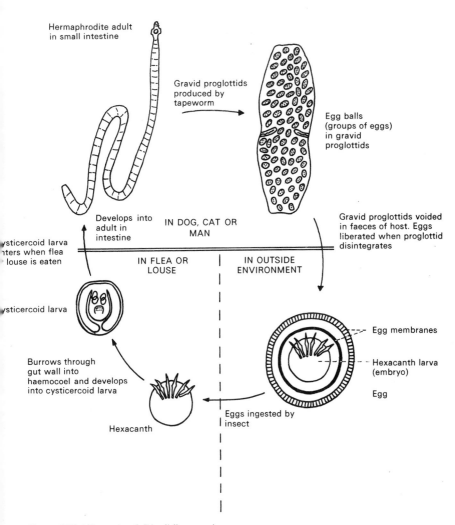

Figure 134 Life cycle of *Dipylidium caninum*.

infected by eating grasshoppers of the genus *Melanoplus*
containing immature stages of the worm.

Habronema microstoma and H. megastoma   *H. microstoma* occurs
in the stomach of equines, as does the closely related *H.*

megastoma. In both worms the larvae are voided in the excreta of the definitive host and are eaten by the maggot larvae of either *Musca domestica* (*H. megastoma*) or *Stomoxys calcitrans* (*H. microstoma*). As the larva pupates so the nematodes reach the infective stage and are passed over to the imago in which they are found in the haemocoel. Within the adult insect the worms pass anteriorly to the head and proboscis, from which they are liberated to be deposited around the mouths of horses when the flies feed in that region. The larvae are subsequently ingested and develop in the stomach of the equines.

Thelazia rhodesii   This parasite is found in the eyes and tear ducts of cattle, sheep and goats in Europe, Africa and Asia, where the intermediate hosts are the muscid flies *Musca larvipara* and *M. convexifrons*. The first-stage larva of the nematode is ingested by the fly when it feeds on the eye secretions of the mammal and the worms migrate through the insect's gut wall to develop to the second- and then third-stage larva in the tissues of the ovarian follicles. Eventually the infective larvae move to the proboscis of the fly and are transferred to a new definitive host when the fly refeeds on eye secretions.

Cestoda

All tapeworms are gut parasites and show variable life histories with animals from many different phyla acting as intermediate hosts. Those which are transmitted by insects, however, share a common life cycle pattern exemplified by *Dipylidium caninum*, described below.

Cestodes parasitic in man

Dipylidium caninum   Although primarily a parasite of cats and dogs this parasite has been recorded from man on many occasions. It is distributed throughout Europe and North America and many other parts of the world, where it is transmitted by various fleas and lice.

When the proglottids become gravid they break away from the strobila of the adult tapeworm and are voided in the faeces of the host. Subsequently these proglottids disintegrate to release their eggs which are then ingested by larval fleas of *Ctenocephalides canis*, *C. felis felis* or *Pulex irritans*, or by the louse *Trichodectes canis*. The ingested eggs hatch in the intestine of the insect and the hexacanth larvae which emerge burrow through the gut wall into the haemocoel where they develop into cysticercoid larvae (Fig. 134) by the time that the flea has become adult. Infection of the definitive host follows the ingestion of insects containing cysticercoids. These are released from the insectan tissues to establish themselves in the alimentary canal of the definitive host, where they grow and mature to become adult tapeworms.

Hymenolepis diminuta   *H. diminuta* occurs in man, mice and rats in most parts of the world. The intermediate hosts of this tapeworm are various moths, for example *Tinea* and *Aglossa* species; beetles, for example *Akis* and *Scaurus* species; earwigs, for example *Anisolabris* species; as well as many species of cockroach, flea and millipede.

Hymenolepis nana   This species is also a gut parasite of man, mice and rats and is found throughout Europe, Africa, Asia, America and Oceania. In rodent infections various fleas and beetles, for example *Tenebrio* and *Tribolium* species, act as intermediate hosts, although in human infections no intermediate host exists and transmission from man to man is direct, with the eggs of the tapeworm being the infective stage.

Cestodes parasitic in non-human hosts
In addition to the tapeworms listed above which affect rodents, cats and dogs, there are two others which deserve mention. They are *Raillietina cesticillus* and *Choanotaenia infundibulum*, both from the small intestine of the fowl and turkey in most parts of the world. Both tapeworms share *Musca domestica* and various beetles as intermediate hosts, although the genera of beetles which act as

transmitters vary in the two species. In *R. cesticillus* the genera *Calathus* and *Amara* are intermediates, while in the case of *C. infundibulum*, *Tribolium* beetles serve the role.

Digenoidea

Usually, the life cycle of a digenoid involves the use of one intermediate host, a mollusc. However, a few species require a second such host which is often an arthropod and which in the species given below is an insect.

Dicrocoelium dendriticum (Fig. 135)   Sheep, goats, pigs, dogs, rabbits and occasionally man and other animals may harbour this parasite in their bile ducts. *D. dendriticum* occurs throughout Europe, North America and Asia and has a snail as its first intermediate host and an ant as its second. In Europe the snail host is usually *Zebrina detrita* while in North America *Cionella lubrica* is the main species involved. As far as second intermediate hosts are concerned, these are *Formica* species with *F. fusca* being common to both Europe and America.

Eggs laid by the fluke are voided from the mammal together with faecal material, and do not hatch until they are ingested by the snail. On hatching the miracidium larvae penetrate the wall of the molluscan gut and migrate to the digestive gland where they develop into sporocyst larvae. These give rise to second generation sporocysts which subsequently develop to cercaria larvae without the intervention of a redia larval stage, normally characteristic of fluke life cycles. The cercariae congregate in the pulmonary chamber of the snail, the mass of larvae being called a slime ball, and such aggregations are expelled from the snail and may be eaten by ants. If ingested by the correct species of ant the cercariae burrow from the gut to the haemocoel and develop into metacercariae. No further development takes place until the ant is eaten by the definitive host, in which case the metacercariae enter the bile duct by way of the intestine and there develop into adult flukes.

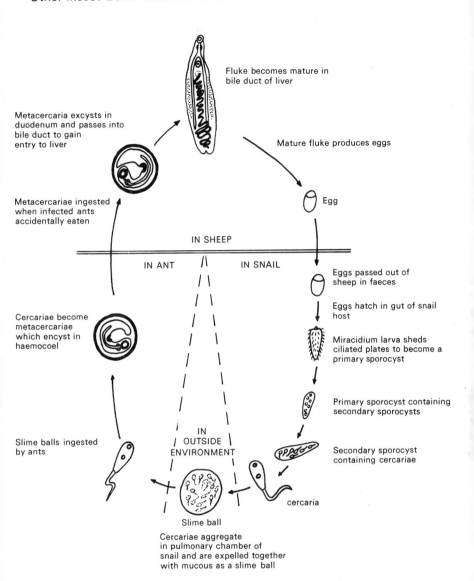

Figure 135 Life cycle of *Dicrocoelium dendriticum*.

Prosthogonimus ovatus   This fluke is found in the oviduct and cloaca of fowl, geese and various wild birds in Europe, Africa and Asia. Two intermediate hosts are required in the life cycle of this trematode. The first of these is a water snail, for example *Bithynia leachi*, and the second is a nymph of a dragonfly of the genus *Libellula*, *Platycnemis* or *Epicordulia*. The avian definitive host is infected by ingesting either the nymph or adult insect.

Eurytrema pancreaticum   *E. pancreaticum* spends its life cycle in a land snail, for example *Bradybaena similaris*, a grasshopper, for example *Conocephalus maculatus*, and sheep, cattle or goats in Asia and South America, and in man in China. In the snail primary and secondary sporocysts develop, the latter giving rise to cercariae which escape on to herbage to be eaten by grasshoppers. Infective metacercariae are found in the haemocoel of the insect and mature in the pancreatic ducts, bile ducts and duodenum of the mammalian host.

Acanthocephala

Adult acanthocephalans, or spiny-headed worms, are found chiefly in aquatic vertebrates, namely fishes and birds, although a few species parasitize mammals. As far as is known, the eggs require to be ingested by an intermediate host, which is usually an arthropod. In this relatively small group of animals only two species will be mentioned, both of which are insect-transmitted.

Macracanthorhynchus hirudinaceus (Fig. 136)   This parasite is found in the small intestine of the pig, and sometimes man, in many countries. Eggs of this worm pass out of the body of the mammal in the faeces and are ingested by beetle larvae, often those of *Melolontha vulgaris*. Within the beetle the eggs hatch and the emergent acanthor larva bores through the gut wall to the haemocoel. Here it develops first to an acanthella larva and then into a cysticanth larva, which is the stage infective to the definitive host. This is transferred when the intermediate host is eaten. In the gut of the final host the cysticanth is activated and attaches to the gut wall by means of its spiny proboscis and matures to the adult stage.

Moniliformis moniliformis   Although this is normally a parasite of rodents it has been reported from human hosts many times. *M. moniliformis* is an intestinal parasite occurring in many parts of the world, including Italy, Sudan, Israel and North America, where various beetles, for example *Blaps* species, and cockroaches, for example *Periplaneta americana*, serve as intermediate hosts. If infected insects gain access to human food then they may be accidentally ingested, with a result that cysticanths will be liberated and adult worms established in the intestine of man.

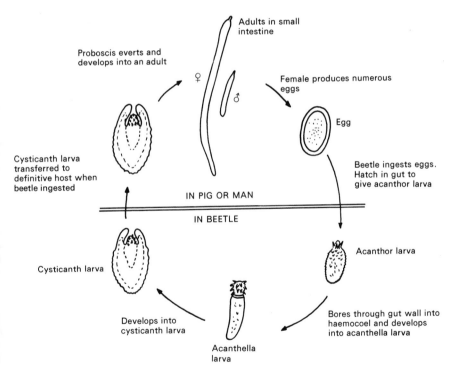

Figure 136 Life cycle of *Macracanthorhynchus hirudinaceus*.

Appendix I

The main orders of insects

In the present text we are concerned with only a few types of insect, but it is important to know where these fit into classificatory schemes. For this reason an abridged version of a classification of the class Insecta is given below, showing the important orders and, where possible, their common names. Orders containing insects of major medical or veterinary importance are marked with an asterisk.

Subclass 1 Apterygota

Insects lacking wings and with slight or no metamorphosis; abdominal appendages in adult in addition to genitalia and cerci.

Order 1 Collembola   (*springtails*)
         2 Thysanura   (*bristletails and silverfish*)
         3 Protura
         4 Diplura

Subclass 2 Pterygota

Insects possessing wings or having secondarily lost them; locomotory abdominal appendages lacking; metamorphosis varied but never slight or absent.

Infraclass 1 Palaeoptera

Insects in which the wings do not fold back over the body when at rest; metamorphosis is gradual (hemimetabolous) and the immature stages (nymphs) are aquatic; wings develop externally—exopterygote condition.

Order   5 Ephemeroptera   (*mayflies*)
       6 Odonata   (*dragonflies*)

Infraclass 2 Polyneoptera
Wings fold back over body when at rest; metamorphosis gradual
(hemimetabolous) and wings develop externally—exopterygote
condition; numerous Malpighian tubules.

Order   7 Plecoptera   (*stoneflies*)
       8 Orthoptera   (*grasshoppers, locusts and crickets*)
       9 Phasmida   (*stick and leaf insects*)
      10 Dermaptera   (*earwigs*)
      11 Embioptera   (*webspinners*)
      12 Dictyoptera   (*cockroaches and mantids*)
      13 Isoptera   (*termites*)

Infraclass 3 Paraneoptera
Wings folded when at rest; metamorphosis gradual
(hemimetabolous) and wings develop outside the body—
exopterygote condition; few Malphighian tubules.

Order 14 Thysanoptera   (*thrips*)
      15 Psocoptera   (*booklice*)
      16 *Mallophaga   (*biting lice*)
      17 *Anoplura   (*sucking lice*)
      18 *Hemiptera   (*bugs*)

Infraclass 4 Oligoneoptera
Wings folded when at rest; metamorphosis complex
(holometabolous) and the immature stage is a larva which differs
markedly from the adult; wings develop inside the body—
endopterygote condition.

Order 19 Coleoptera   (*beetles*)
      20 Megaloptera   (*alderflies*)
      21 Mecoptera   (*scorpionflies*)
      22 Neuroptera   (*lacewings and antlions*)
      23 Raphidioptera   (*snakeflies*)
      24 Trichoptera   (*caddisflies*)

25 Lepidoptera   (*butterflies and moths*)
26 *Siphonaptera   (*fleas*)
27 Hymenoptera   (*bees, wasps and ants*)
28 *Diptera   (*true flies*)
29 Strepsiptera   (*stylopids*)

Appendix II

Outline classifications of the Protozoa, Platyhelminthes, Nematoda, Acanthocephala and various microorganisms
The object of this section is to place the pathogenic organisms mentioned in the text into a scheme of classification so that the relationships between forms can be seen, and to help the reader when referring to other books. Complete classifications are not attempted here for they are both lengthy and complex.

1 **Phylum PROTOZOA**
Small organisms, the bodies of which are nucleated and built on an acellular plan.

Subphylum Sarcomastigophora
Amoeboid and flagellate protozoans with monomorphic nuclei; spores absent; sexual reproduction, if present, involves syngamy.
Superclass Mastigophora
  Vegetative stages move using flagella.
Class Phytomastigophorea
  Mostly free-living, plant-like flagellates; chromatophores present or secondarily lost, but with the relationship to pigmented forms remaining apparent.
Class Zoomastigophorea
  Free-living or parasitic; chromatophores absent and not closely related to pigmented forms.
  Order Kinetoplastida (*Trypanosoma, Leishmania*)

Superclass Opalinata
 Numerous short flagella arranged in longitudinal rows; two to
 many monomorphic nuclei.
Superclass Sarcodina
 Pseudopodia present for feeding and locomotion.
Class Rhizopodea
 Pseudopodia lobose, filose or reticulose.
 Order Amoebida (*Entamoeba*)
Class Actinopodea
 Pelagic or sessile forms with pseudopodia radiating from a
 spherical body.

Subphylum Sporozoa
Spores typically present which lack a polar filament; all parasitic;
cilia and flagella absent except for microgametes of some forms;
nuclei monomorphic; sexual reproduction, if present, involves
syngamy.
Class Telosporea
 Spores present; locomotion by gliding and body flexion;
 pseudopodia, if present, are for feeding only.
Subclass Gregarinia
 Mature trophozoites large and extracellular; parasites of the
 gut and body cavity of invertebrates.
Subclass Coccidia
 Mature trophozoites small and typically intracellular.
 Order Eucoccida
    Suborder Adeleina   (*Hepatozoon*)
              Eimeriina   (*Lankesterella*)
              Haemosporina   (*Plasmodium, Haemoproteus,
                               Leucocytozoon, Hepatocystis*)
Class Piroplasmea
 Amoeboid parasites of vertebrate erythrocytes (*Babesia*).

Subphylum Cnidospora
Spores with polar filaments; all parasitic.

Subphylum Ciliophora

Simple or compound cilia present during the life cycle; nuclei dimorphic; homothetigenic binary fission; sexual reproduction involving conjugation, cytogamy and autogamy (*Balantidium*).

2 Phylum PLATYHELMINTHES

Normally dorso-ventrally flattened, unsegmented hermaphrodite worms which lack a body cavity; respiratory and circulatory systems are absent and excretory system is composed of flame cells.

Class Turbellaria

Mainly non-parasitic having a ciliated outer body covering; parasitic species do not affect man and his domestic stock.

Class Digenoidea

Body composed of a single region, that is not subdivided as in Cestodes; oral and ventral suckers present for attachment to the host; gut is bifurcated and has a mouth but no anus; digenoids are nearly always hermaphrodite, the only exception being the dioecious schistosomes; life cycle involves one or more intermediate hosts; endoparasites.

Family Dicrocoeliidae   (*Dicrocoelium, Eurytrema*)
       Plagiorchidae   (*Prosthogonimus*)

Class Monogenoidea

Similar to the Digenoidea, but with a complex posterior attachment organ (opisthaptor) equipped with hooks, clamps and suckers and with a life history involving only one host; do not affect man and domesticated animals; mainly ectoparasitic.

Class Cestoda

Usually with bodies consisting of serially repeated units called proglottids, each containing one or more sets of hermaphrodite reproductive organs; gut is absent and the scolex is equipped with suckers and sometimes hooks for attachment; endoparasitic.

Order Cyclophyllidea

Family Davaineidae   (*Raillietina*)

Dilepididae   (*Dipylidium, Choanotaenia*)
Hymenolepididae   (*Hymenolepis*)
Taeniidae   (*Taenia, Echinococcus*)

3 Phylum ACANTHOCEPHALA

Cylindrical worms with a retractable proboscis equipped with
spines; dioecious; no gut; life cycle involves an intermediate
host (*Macracanthorynchus, Moniliformis*).

4 Phylum NEMATODA

Cylindrical, unsegmented pseudocoelomates; circular in cross-
section; body invested by a cuticle and the body wall composed
of longitudinal muscle only.

Order Ascaroidea   (*Ascaris*)
        Strongyloidea   (*Ancylostoma, Necator*)
        Spiruroidea   (*Thelazia, Habronema, Hartertia,
                         Spirocerca, Gongylonema, Acuaria*)
        Filaroidea   (*Onchocerca, Wuchereria, Brugia,
                         Setaria, Dipetalonema, Mansonella, Loa,
                         Dirofilaria*)
        Trichuroidea   (*Trichuris*)
        Oxyuroidea   (*Enterobius, Subulura*)

5 MICROORGANISMS

Bacteria

These are microscopic organisms, some of which are harmful to
other forms of life, which produce resistant spores. The acellular
body does not possess a nucleus. No classification of bacteria
will be entered into here except for the naming based on the
shape and grouping formations.

1 *Shape*

    (a) bacillus — rod-shaped
    (b) coccus — spherical
    (c) spirillum — spiral-shaped
    (d) vibrio — kidney-shaped

2 *Grouping*
    for example   coccus   o

                      diplococcus (two cocci)   ∞

                      streptococcus (chain of cocci)

                      staphylococcus (group of cocci)

Rickettsiae and related organisms

These are small, rod-shaped, spherical or pleomorphic micro-organisms living and multiplying in living tissues. Three groups are recognized, viz. Rickettsiaceae, Bartonellaceae and Chlamydozoaceae, two of which concern us in the present context.

1 *Rickettsiaceae* (*Rickettsiae*)
    Mostly symbionts of arthropods, but some are transferrable to man and other animals causing pathogenic conditions. The pathogenic forms affecting man and higher animals are divided into four genera:
    (a) *Rickettsia*—for example *R. prowazekii*; tick- and insect-transmitted.
    (b) *Coxiella*—one species only, *C. burnetii*, producing Q-fever; tick-borne.
    (c) *Cowdria*—one species only, *C. ruminantium*, producing heart-water fever of domestic stock; transmitted by ticks.
    (d) *Neorickettsia*—one species only, *N. helmintheca*, producing salmon poisoning in salmon-eating mammals.

2 *Bartonellaceae*
    Pleomorphic; parasitize the erythrocytes and sometimes the reticulo-endothelial system of vertebrates. Four genera are recognized:
    (a) *Bartonella*—for example *B. bacilliformis*, producing bartonellosis in man.
    (b) *Haemobartonella*—for example *H. canis* of dogs; method of transmission not known but haematophagous insects may be involved.
    (c) *Grahamella*—rod-like bodies in erythrocytes of moles and other animals.

(d) *Eperythrozoon*—exact systematic position as yet undetermined; minute forms on the surface of erythrocytes and in the plasma, for example, *E. wenyoni* of cattle; lice may be involved in transmission.

Viruses (Virales)
Always pathogenic; minute particles of deoxyribosenucleic acid (DNA) or ribosenucleic acid (RNA) contained within a protein envelope. The arboviruses are contained within this group and their classification is discussed in the text.

Spirochaetes (Spirochaetales)
These parasites are motile and filamentous, with the body thrown into many spirals (e.g. *Borrelia* and *Treponema*); often pathogenic and transmitted by ticks and insects.

Further reading

The following list is intended as a guide so that the reader can pursue the various subjects further. In turn, these texts will direct the reader to more advanced literature, including research publications.

General insectan biology
Chapman, R. F. (1969). *The Insects*. English Universities Press. London.
Imms, A. D. (1957). *A General Textbook of Entomology*. Methuen. London.
Wigglesworth, V. B. (1965). *The Principles of Insect Physiology*. Methuen. London.

General parasitology
Chandler, A. C., and Read, C. P. (1961). *Introduction to Parasitology*. Wiley. New York.
Faust, E. C., and Russell, P. F. (1970). *Craig and Faust's Clinical Parasitology*. Kimpton. London.
Lapage, G. (1963). *Animals Parasitic in Man*. Dover. New York.
Lapage, G. (1968). *Veterinary Parasitology*. Oliver & Boyd. Edinburgh and London.
Rothschild, M., and Clay, T. (1952). *Fleas, Flukes and Cuckoos*. Collins New Naturalist. London.
Smyth, J. D. (1962). *Introduction to Animal Parasitology*. English Universities Press. London.
Soulsby, E. J. L. (1968). *Helminths, Arthropods and Protozoa of Domesticated Animals*. Baillière, Tindall & Cassell. London.

Parasitic insects
Askew, R. R. (1971). *Parasitic Insects*. Heinemann. London.

Bates, M. (1949). *The Natural History of Mosquitoes.* Macmillan. New York.

Buxton, P. A. (1939). *The Louse.* Arnold. London.

Buxton, P. A. (1955). *The Natural History of Tsetse Flies.* Lewis. London.

Clements, A. N. (1963). *The Physiology of Mosquitoes.* Pergamon. Oxford.

Glasgow, J. P. (1963). *The Distribution and Abundance of Tsetse.* Pergamon. Oxford.

Leclercq, M. (1969). *Entomological Parasitology—the Relations between Entomology and the Medical Sciences.* Pergamon. Oxford.

Mattingley, P. F. (1969). *The Biology of Mosquito-borne Disease.* Allen & Unwin. London.

Smart, J. (1965). *A Handbook for the Identification of Insects of Medical Importance.* British Museum (Natural History). London.

Snodgrass, R. E. (1943). *The Feeding Apparatus of Biting and Sucking Insects Affecting Man and Animals.* Smithsonian Miscellaneous Collections. Vol. 104, No. 7.

Pathogens carried by insects

Baker, J. R. (1969). *Parasitic Protozoa.* Hutchinson. London.

Faust, E. C., and Russell, P. F. (1970). *Craig and Faust's Clinical Parasitology.* Kimpton. London.

Garnham, P. C. C. (1966). *Malaria Parasites.* Blackwell. Oxford.

Hoare, C. A. (1971). *The Trypanosomes of Mammals.* Blackwell. Oxford.

Lapage, G. (1963). *Animals Parasitic in Man.* Dover. New York.

Manwell, R. D. (1968). *Introduction to Protozoology.* Dover. New York.

Soulsby, E. J. L. (1968). *Helminths, Arthropods and Protozoa of Domesticated Animals.* Baillière, Tindall & Cassell. London.

Vickerman, K., and Cox, F. E. G. (1967). *The Protozoa.* Murray. London.

Watson, J. M. (1960). *Medical Helminthology.* Baillière, Tindall & Cox. London.

Index